Bear With Me

PLAYS BY DIANE FLACKS

Myth Me (1992)

By a Thread (1994)

Gravity Calling (1994)

Random Acts (1999)

SIBS (2001)
(*With Richard Greenblatt*)

Bear With Me

What they don't tell you about pregnancy and new motherhood

DIANE FLACKS

M&S

Library and Archives Canada Cataloguing in Publication

Flacks, Diane
    Bear with me : what they don't tell you about pregnancy and new motherhood / Diane Flacks.

ISBN 0-7710-4764-9

1. Flacks, Diane.   2. Pregnant women – Biography.
3. Pregnancy – Popular works.   4. Pregnancy – Humor.   I. Title.

RG525.F55 2005   618.2'0092   C2004-906724-9

We acknowledge the financial support of the Government of Canada through the Book Publishing Industry Development Program and that of the Government of Ontario through the Ontario Media Development Corporation's Ontario Book Initiative. We further acknowledge the support of the Canada Council for the Arts and the Ontario Arts Council for our publishing program.

Typeset in Bembo by M&S, Toronto
Printed and bound in Canada

This book is printed on 50% post-consumer waste recycled paper.

McClelland & Stewart Ltd.
The Canadian Publishers
481 University Avenue
Toronto, Ontario
M5G 2E9
www.mcclelland.com

1 2 3 4 5   09 08 07 06 05

To Janis Purdy and Eli Purdy-Flacks

———●———

Some names have been changed in order to
protect privacy . . . or because I've forgotten them.

And the angel said to Abraham, "I will surely return to you at this time next year, and behold Sarah your wife will have a son."... Now Sarah and Abraham were old, well on in years; the manner of women had ceased to be with Sarah. And Sarah laughed.... Then God said to Abraham, "Why is it that Sarah laughed, saying Shall I in truth bear a child, though I have aged?"... Sarah denied it, saying, "I did not laugh."... But God said, "No, you laughed indeed."

— Genesis 18:10–15

Contents

Acknowledgements

Writing is often about finding the little gems that the universe drops in your path. And stealing them. Thanks to all the women who shared their stories, and the strangers whose stories I overheard. You are doing a service to other new parents, so please don't sue.

Huge gratitude to the team at McClelland & Stewart and especially to Elizabeth Kribs, my editor, for her graceful and insightful advice. Also for seeking me out, a brain-addled new mom, after reading a short article that I wrote about sex and pregnancy in *NOW* magazine. Thank you Alice Klein at *NOW* magazine for asking me to write the original article. Thank you Janis, for letting me tattle about our sex life. Special acknowledgement to Rita Silvan at *ELLE* magazine for allowing me to use excerpts from two articles written for the December 2001 and May 2002 editions of *ELLE Canada*.

Huge gratitude and admiration to my mother, Lily Flacks, and my father, Cyril Flacks, whose love, joy, wisdom, and sense of fun have made our lives so rich. Thanks for all the input from my honest, whipsmart sister, Laura Flacks-Narrol, mother of Jordan, and my big brother, Daniel Flacks.

Special thanks to my kind and generous mother-in-law, Doris Purdy.

Thanks to the core group of pals from whom I leeched information, and who encouraged me along the way: Netty Kruger,

Ruth Marshall, Victoria Jakowenko. Also thanks to Sara Booth, Ilana Lewis, Ellie Harvie, Todd Narrol, Kelly Flacks, Waneta Storms, Dr. David Greenberg, Alisa Palmer, Ann-Marie MacDonald, Ian Purdy, Alan Purdy, Ann Purdy, Patricia Rozema, Leslie Barber, Cyd Israel, Shari Goldberg, Joyce Coombs, Zoe Neuman, Andrea Fogel, Wendel Meldrum, Odette McCarthy, Lisa Silverman, Lynne Harvey, Leslie Lester, Richard Greenblatt, Bruce McCulloch, Robin Severin, Sandra Ferguson, Fiona Highet, Sasha Padron and Kathryn Beet from the Yoga Space, Michelle Rival, Bev Cooper, Maria Del Mar, Sass Jordan, Rochelle Strauss, Naomi Moscoe, Leslie Schwartz, Chrisanthe Michaelides, Lori Smith, Kathryn Greenwood, Lara Ellis, Dr. Rochelle Schwartz, Jane Ford, Wendy Fraser, Michele Landsberg, Judy Rebick, Gail Singer. Also thanks to my writing agents at Great North Artist Management: Rena Zimmerman and Shain Jaffe.

My midwife moms-group pals: Nancy Paris, Aara Amey, Mary Young, Diana Dampier, and Dina Ladd and Mary Gellatly. My yoga moms-group chickies: Michelle Rothstein, Nancy Friedland, Hannah Fowley, Sarah MacKenzie, Lisa Lev, Rosie Little, Ilana Lewis. Prim Pemberton's writing group, who saw a few chapters very early on and provided affirmation, experience, and concise advise: Kate Story, Phillipa Domville, Peter Sanders, Ilene Cummings, Rachel Giese, Annie Jacobson, and Guy Ratchford. Our uber-tenant and friend Dawn Whitwell for reading early chapters, laughing, crying, and helping to spice up some jokes.

Special kudos and thanks to David Gale, and to Ruthy Gale.

Mostly to Janis, my partner, whose candour, wit, bravery, and maternal innovation made this possible. All my heart.

Finally Eli, the sweetest, cutest angel in the world. *K'nein a hora.*

Introduction

*Before I was pregnant, when I heard people say that having a
child changes your life and becomes your focus, I'd think,
Wow, you must not have much of a career.*

I was not only flippant, I was clueless. I would go to friends'
houses who had kids and lounge about while *they* made *me*
tea. I did not bring a hot meal, or hold their baby while they
bathed and had a nap. I didn't understand that you shouldn't call
the parents of a newborn and say, "We haven't seen you guys in a
while. What's up?" And invite them to go to a movie in an hour.
In effect, torturing them with an offer of a social engagement they
can only dream about.

"Motherhood is one of the only things in life you simply can't
describe to anyone who hasn't gone through it. Climbing
Everest you can describe and people could get a feel for it.
Until you empathetically connect with the parenting experi-
ence, it cannot be explained. You can only know by doing it."
– Rona, mother of one

I

Sure enough, as soon as I got pregnant, it was as if someone had placed mother-lenses on my eyes – everything was now viewed through them, and refracted into beautiful, disorienting rainbows of new life. Now, I can't go back to seeing the world as I had before. I don't really miss it, though. I can't remember where I put my purse, much less what life used to be like P.B. (pre-baby).

WHY? – WHY *NOT*?
I wrote this book for two reasons: 1) Because moms need to talk, and 2) because people want us to shut up.

Can We Talk?!
When I was pregnant I realized there was so much I was experiencing that I had not seen portrayed in mainstream representations of pregnancy. There seemed to be a deliberate, nice, polished image that predominated. And I had messy, awkward questions like: "Okay, is it my imagination, or are my pubes getting longer? Am I crazy, or are my nails growing at an alarming rate? And is it possible to cut them with anything other than a blowtorch." (The answers to the above are: yes, yes, and try a hacksaw.)

So I joined moms groups (a handful or strangers who are as shut-in with their new needy baby as you are and with whom you have nothing else in common). I harassed my midwife with questions, browsed Internet chat rooms. I wished that I had more books to read; and I sent the titles of the good ones on to everyone I knew who was even thinking of trying to conceive. I realized that there was a dearth of information on the real stuff, the nitty-gritty, the *shit* that I hoped I was not alone in experiencing.

One day in my son's first year, I dropped in to a dinner party and got swept into a conversation with two women while he ran around screeching joyfully and trying to ingest carpet fluff. I mentioned that I was writing this book. They looked at me and shook their heads.

"I loved being pregnant," said one. Her clipped tone implying, Why would you write a book about it? Here's my book: *Piece. Of. Cake.*

"Me too, I loved it," concurred the second.

I knew better by this point than to say anything.

There was a pause.

"Now, my *birth* experience," burst the first woman, "that was a horror show."

"Disaster," piped in the second.

"I was hooked up to every tube there was. I had every intervention."

"*My* first came out backwards so I thought she had hair on her face like a monkey."

And then the confessions really got going:

"I put on fifty pounds!"

"*I* ended up at one-ninety!"

We continued boisterously spilling the beans, while my son spun around singing, "Bus! bus! bus!" and a seven-year-old boy bounced a soccer ball off of his head, assuring me, "He likes it!"

Meanwhile, the men in the room slowly inched away from us and toward the spanakopita.

The Shut-up Response

Why is it that we know more about Viagra than Diclectin (an anti-nausea drug safe to use while pregnant)? Why do we have more films, books, plays, TV shows, psychological nomenclature, and buzz words for a man's "midlife crisis" than for what happens to a relationship after a baby arrives? Why do we have a thesaurus full of words for "jacking off," but no accurate descriptors of the pain of labour?

I recently heard a radio interview with singer/songwriter Nelly Furtado. The disc jockey was commenting on Furtado's new status as a mother. He said something to the effect of "You seem so relaxed about it. When Céline Dion had a baby, it was like she invented motherhood. Like no one had ever done this before."

Well, excuse Céline for talking about one of the single most important experiences in her life. We'll all be quiet now so you can get back to your story about the history of the toque. There is a sense that people want us moms to keep quiet. I don't know about you, but that makes me want to talk. Loud and clear.

Feminist writer Naomi Wolf, author of *The Beauty Myth*, caused a frenzy when she appeared on *The Oprah Winfrey Show* to promote her recently published book *Misconceptions*. The show stirred up so much controversy that she had to do a followup appearance a few days later. *Oprah* allowed Naomi and other women to give voice to some heartwrenching experiences that they had previously kept to themselves. Everything from breast-feeding pain to lack of sex drive was discussed. This made some people very angry. Particularly other mothers.

One audience member stood up and said, "I am a mother and damn proud of it. I loved every second of motherhood, including labour and my episiotomy." The unspoken comment was "So shut up."

Whose agenda are we promoting by keeping the details, awesome and painful, of motherhood secret? By shutting up and being cheerful, compliant good girls? Why must we judge each other for our different responses? Does our culture pressure women to be quiet about the realities of motherhood so that we will accept our lot and not push for more help, more involvement, more power? Although this book's aim isn't to answer social ills, it hopes to release other moms . . . to bitch about them too.

After all, it's part of human nature to want to tell stories. Telling and retelling particularly stinging or profound anecdotes allows distance, embellishment, and humour to make them easier to cope with. Most importantly, storytelling fosters a sense of connection with others. This book is written in the hopes that these "battle stories" might resonate with other women. Spark in them the desire to speak loudly about their experiences; to continue a rollicking, fierce, and free conversation about our lives.

HOW I GATHERED MATERIAL

My primary method of gathering material for this book was connected to my aim in writing it: I talked to other women. Some of the quotes from myself and my partner come from our journals, and some are from e-mails to and from friends. I read other women's accounts. I spoke to midwives, to moms groups, dads, and I received confessions from perfect strangers. I talked to my wonderful family, and especially my funny and compassionate mother, Lily, and mother-in-law, Doris. I picked the brain of my patient, sultry partner, Janis.

Although some people in this book have had their names and story details changed, I've tried to be as true to the spirit of my own and other women's experiences as I can. The mind is an imperfect sifter, so please forgive any inaccuracies.

THE GAY THING

Just one word on The Gay Thing. People have asked me how being a lesbian has affected my parenting. I am tempted to say, "I'm too busy chasing a toddler to know."

In getting pregnant, being a lesbian had a big impact, of course. As you can imagine, it's not as straightforward (pardon the pun) as with heterosexual couples. Although, we did share many similar hurdles, as you'll see in the first chapter. My partner and I found that we had a lot in common with heterosexual couples who were having trouble conceiving and who needed assistance with fertility. I often kibitzed with straight women about the exorbitant cost of ovulation kits, and the loss of romanticism that occurs when you have to try to conceive on a schedule.

When I became pregnant, being gay didn't matter one bit. Hot, huge, and cranky comes in all orientations. Now that I'm a mom,

I just feel lucky that my partner is a person who is wholly committed to an equitable relationship of caregiving to our child. Understanding, patience, willingness to take on full responsibility for the raising of the child, and not seeing your role strictly as "helping" the mother are all key factors in being a good partner and parent, and should have nothing to do with gender.

Mind you, it's been a bonus that Janis can totally relate to bloating, mood swings, odd bodily leakages, and spontaneous bouts of tears and laughter. Welcome to motherhood.

1

Getting Knocked Up

"Honey, could you hurry up, Survivor
is on in three minutes."

Many couples experience a renewed sexual abandon when they try to conceive. No more pills, messy condoms, or slippery diaphragms. They just do it like teenagers: reckless, dirty, wild. Everywhere and anywhere. Because, they assure their friends, they have to.

It's all very funny until you go away with said couple on a camping trip and you open the back of their van to look for a Balance Bar and instead see a feat of balance that you will sadly never erase from your memory.

This kind of romantic fervour can only be sustained for a few months. After which time it becomes, "Sweetie, could you finish up, the dog wants out."

THE BIG DECISION

My partner and I are dedicated to our careers. As a writer and actor, I have been known to laboriously workshop new plays deep into the night, for four hundred dollars a week. Before tax. Although I've been fortunate enough to write for and act in half-a-dozen Canadian TV series, creating intimate theatre is what I love best.

Janis works for a non-profit agency. She has worked with street youth, battered women, gay kids. When she creates a project, she becomes consumed by it. She does it right.

In the first years of our relationship, I was constantly wrestling with both of our super-agendas. Trying to carve out some time just for us. It was tough enough competing with street kids for Janis's attention, I sure didn't want to throw a baby into the mix.

I was thirty-three when Janis really pressed the issue of one of us getting pregnant. Thirty-three is how old Christ was reported to be when he was crucified. I referred to thirty-three as my "bite me" year. I felt old enough, and professionally experienced enough, to respond to questions like, "Can you write us a few sketches for free and then we'll decide if we want to hire you?" with, "Can you *bite* me?" The last thing I wanted was to sacrifice my hard-earned veteran status by taking myself out of the professional milieu for a few years.

Plus, I was afraid of babies, and intimidated by children – with their truthful, open faces and their too-honest assessments of adults. "Why are you acting so silly?" was a common question children posed to me, and I had no answer for it.

Like many people in their thirties, I had finally let go of my angst. I'd kicked much of my needy, poetry-writing, people-pleasing tendencies to the curb. I was the most balanced, reasonable, and emotionally settled I had been in my life. So for sure, *I* was not interested in getting pregnant. I did not need messy hormones fogging things up for me.

Not to mention what it might do to my body. At that time, I was in the best shape of my life. I was, as my doctor put it, "ripped."

Imagine if I got pregnant! The Flacks hips-and-ass gene would finally stalk me down and spread itself out, making me unmarketable in our thin-obsessed media.

I tried explaining all of this to Janis, but for all of my fears, she had sensible counter-arguments. This was wildly irritating. So, I tried this old line: "Don't you want me to agree that we should have a child when *I* really want it? This is not something you'd want me to do just to make *you* happy, is it?"

It worked. I was in the clear.

Around the same time I got a stupendous career break. I was approached to help create, write, and act in a Canadian TV series – with a decent budget!

I started to write the pilot, with much creative help and input from the producers. It began smoothly, but the calm didn't last. Accompanying the bigger budget were more demands and opinions. At one point, I was tempted to walk away from the project, unnerved by the prospect that this edgy, fragile dramedy could become *Yes, Dear.* As shooting began, and compromises were made, I felt split down the middle. I wanted success and money, and was terribly grateful for the break, but I was deeply unhappy. I couldn't sleep. I came home in knots and in tears. I tried to be funny.

One night I looked around, and in my best Peggy Lee, I warbled, "Is that all there is?" Is this unstable, somewhat ridiculous career really enough? There must be more to life.

I woke Janis.

"Let's do it," I whispered.

She opened her eyes a crack, and flinched. She didn't know exactly who she would be greeting each morning: Dopey, Hopey, or Mopey. She cagily ventured, "Do what?"

"Let's have that baby."

She felt my forehead for fever, and then we started scheming.

SEARCHING FOR SEEDS

Our plan was that Janis would carry the child, and I would take care of her. I'd wrap my arms around her and our babe. I'd be their champion, and our love would form a shield to protect us.

But love could not a baby make. We had the eggs, now we needed the seed.

Good pals in a similar situation had gone to a fertility clinic to find an anonymous sperm donor. The process of using the sperm clinic is fairly straightforward. The biological mom gets checked out to make sure that all her pipes are clean, that her fertility won't be an issue. Then she looks through tons of donor profiles, often on the Internet. These profiles include detailed medical and personality information, and an indication whether the donor would allow your child to meet him when s/he turns eighteen – knock on wood. (Or as my mother would say, "All's well, *k'nein a hora*, ptoo ptoo, you should only live to have a teenager, and they should only be good as gold and not sell drugs.")

Our friends Rose and Charmaine scanned the profiles of hundreds of men. They were looking for a clean medical history and well-rounded hobbies:

> "We immediately nixed anyone who listed 'bodybuilding' or 'hunting.' We narrowed it down to fifty men. Then we each went through the files on our own and chose our favourite. We both picked the same guy."

Once the donor is picked, the biological mother is tested to see when she's ovulating. This takes the form of blood tests, very early in the morning. When her surge of hormones indicates that it's time, she comes to the clinic and she is inseminated with "washed sperm." I imagined tiny clotheslines with microscopic clothes pegs holding millions of sperm in place as they drip-dried in the breeze.

Clinically speaking, washing sperm means that the sperm is separated from the seminal fluid. This is also referred to as "spinning the sperm" – which does *not* mean that the little guys sweat it out on itty-bitty bikes in the testicular gym.

After the sperm is washed or spun, it is injected directly into the woman's uterus through a long, intimidating-looking pipette at the end of a syringe.

Sperm is stored frozen, and unlike those fish sticks that are crystallizing in your freezer at this very moment, it can stay frozen for years. A couple that we know had a child with sperm from a clinic, then had another one with the same sperm sample seven years later. According to the Web site of a local sperm bank, ReproMed Limited, sperm has "little or no loss per cent cryosurvival after 25 years of storage at -196°C."

A single mom we know from New York was inseminated with frozen sperm for months, at the cost of thousands of dollars, but she couldn't get pregnant. In determining the donor, she had painstakingly picked the most intellectually gifted man in the bunch of wankers. After continued failed attempts, the nurses at the clinic encouraged her to go with a different donor. Apparently, Eggy can be choosy. The ovum sometimes simply doesn't jive with a particular sperm. The clinic staff recommended a guy whom they all loved. A real sweetie. Sure, he was an Orthodox Jew and my friend was a Reformist feminist. Okay, he wasn't that bright. Fine, he had large farmer's hands and prominent facial features, but, the staff assured her, a nicer guy, you could not find ejaculating anywhere. My pal went for it. She got pregnant the next month. As it turns out, her son is a bit of a genius. With big hands.

Although I was tempted by the notion of just us two becoming three, in the end we both desired a known donor for our child.

Now how to find the right one?

FINDING DADDY

Would we want someone who'd simply slip us their DNA? Who'd just want to see the child at Christmas? Or who'd want to co-parent? I was pretty sure the latter option wasn't for me. Parenting with someone I love desperately would be challenging enough. I couldn't imagine trying to share custody with someone I kinda didn't mind once I'd had a few.

Then I thought of David. Curly-haired, gregarious, bright-eyed David Gale is an actor/writer, singer/dancer, and all-around schtick-maestro. He scored a television hit as the host of *Loving Spoonfuls*, a show where he cooked and kibitzed with different grandmothers each week. The series was moving and funny, and David handled the unpredictability with a wink and aplomb.

David and I first met in the late 1980s, when many of us in the alternative theatre community wrote and performed our own plays – basically for each other. David and I were drawn to drunk-enly dirty-dance together at theatre parties. Probably because we were both Jewish and liked Technotronic. One night we vowed, through slurps of warm beer, that since we both had green eyes, if we weren't married by the time we were thirty-five, we would get together and have little "Fl-ales."

So, fifteen years after that plastered promise, at the age of thirty-four, I looked up David's number in an old address book. I hadn't seen him in a while. I left a message on his answering machine: "Hi, David, long time no speak. Don't know if you remember the 'Fl-ales' idea, but my partner and I are thinking of having a child with a known donor. Are you interested in talking to us?"

He called right back.

"It's what I've been wanting all my life," he said.

Okay, that scared us. We didn't want someone wanting this too much.

THE CONTRACT

But we really liked David. So, over the next year or so, David, Janis, and I met bimonthly with a professional mediator to see if it was possible to forge out a parenting contract that suited the three of us. We were ignorant of parenting requirements, the law, or our future, but we had enthusiasm. In short, we were just like most new parents.

We looked around for queer family models that might complement us. Denise and Devorah have a child with Steve. He sees him once every two weeks. Steve doesn't provide financial support. The mothers form the nuclear family unit. They have all the decision-making authority and do all the day-to-day parenting. The child calls Steve Dad, and Steve acts like one – he's not the "treat guy," he disciplines when needed. The moms are called "custodial parents" and Steve is called an "access parent."

We started negotiating using this queerified custodial/access model as a basis. The mediation sessions started out well but became fractious. Our open-hearted notion of "more family equals more love and isn't that what children really need?" melted in the face of the details. We tried to cover everything from vacations to birthdays to grandparents. Each subject brought up strong, visceral reactions. And no one had even got knocked up yet!

As much as I was charmed by David and knew he was a loving person, his enthusiasm made me uneasy. I worried that he actually wanted to co-parent. Janis and I desired to be free to raise this child ourselves, within our relationship in our home. Plus we wanted a known Dad who would have a special, separate relationship with him or her. We wanted it all.

We approached David with our suspicions. He assured us that he was pushing hard because he was acting like he would in any "negotiation." He reiterated that what we wanted was indeed what he wanted. He loved his lifestyle, his career, and did not seek to co-parent. But he wished to be called Daddy and to meet parental expectations during his time with the child. *He* wanted it all.

In the end, we all caved a bit, and signed our contract. We celebrated by going out for Indian food. I watched Janis and David shmooze with the waiter. My hands shook. My stomach churned. Who was this person whose genes would be mingling with my partner's?

My tip for anyone entering into a similar negotiation is this: Do not try to create a good fit. This process is not about how well you can "make things work" between you.

Be uncompromising about details that mean a lot to you, and articulate all your expectations, no matter how obvious they may seem. If you don't hash it out now, the areas that you concede on in the spirit of "good negotiation" may rear their heads later. Be patient. A good match is worth the fight. It certainly was in our case. And we have our magnificent son, Eli, to show for it!

Like with all parents, our challenges, joys, and conflicts continue to knock us all off our pins on a regular basis. The very first challenge was a doozy.

THE FIRST TIME: "What exactly do two women *do* in bed (to make a baby)?"

According to my research (watching TV), there are people who would be very interested to know how Janis, David, and I did it.

One of the bonuses in discovering that I was a lesbian was the assumption that I would not have to have very much to do with sperm in my lifetime. Suddenly I had to become an aficionado.

Let me say straight up, we did not have sex with our donor.

Phew. David would hang out downstairs in our living room and watch some Italian porn (the background music of which is indelibly burned into my cervical cortex). He had a sterile cup into which he would aim his biological material at the conclusion of viewing said porn. (Is this clear enough?!)

We would wait upstairs in our bedroom, pillows propped precariously under Janis's bum. He would knock on the door and hand off the cup. I would take it, and pour it into a syringe, trying not to inhale. (Even you straight couples have to admit there's a definite tang.) I would then inject the surprisingly viscous contents of the syringe into Janis, aiming for her cervix as well as I could.

The first time we inseminated, Janis and I went to David's funky, meticulously decorated west-end apartment. Janis and I went into his bedroom and bobbed about on the waterbed. We listened to Aretha Franklin. We held each other tenderly, gazing lovingly into each other's eyes, trying not to be distracted by David's collection of Judaica.

After the insemination, we got into our car and started for home. Janis drove, trying not to grind the gears or shake herself up too much, which was tough because I was clinging to her shifting arm, sobbing sloppily. It finally hit me that, after a year of talk, we were really doing it. We were really trying to make a baby. I didn't realize it at the time, but besides being moved by the gravity of our undertaking, I was mourning the loss of our youth. Our Petra Pan, forever-young days were behind us. And something in me was very, very angry about that. This part of me secretly hoped the insemination wouldn't take. As my mother would say, be careful what you wish for.

THE LONG ROAD

What is it about guys and size? Every single time we inseminated, David would nudge me with his elbow and whisper, "Pretty big cupful today, huh?" I hate to be breaking it to him sort of publicly like this, but it was basically the same amount each time: two and a half to three cc's. A healthy amount, sure, yes: big, bigger, biggest!

As we kept at it, it became less and less of a romantic or emotional procedure. And definitely not sexual. My doctor told us that if Janis had an orgasm, it would help our chances. The doctor drew us a little cartoon to explain the science of it. The uterus contracts during orgasm so that the tip of the cervix dips into the back of the vagina; in effect, slurping up any sperm that's pooling there. So, heads up, ladies, you need to come too.

After trying for about six months with no success, I broached my methodology with my doctor. Was there anything I, the lowly syringe girl, could do to make this take? He suggested that instead of sucking the sperm into the syringe, I pour it in the syringe, gently, so as not to traumatize any of the little guys.

Sounded good to me. The next night I was ready. I grabbed the cup and, in a chivalrous attempt at maintaining a mood, I shielded Janis from the view. I painstakingly poured into the syringe. I was concentrating so hard on the pouring that I didn't remember to block the other end of the syringe. Everything spilled out. It moved so fast, I couldn't stop it.

"Oops," I gasped, as I watched it all plop to the ground.

"Oops what?" Janis craned her neck to look.

"I dropped it."

"*It?*"

"Yeah, it, all of it. It spilled. Peuw!"

"Can you pick it up?"

I didn't want to touch it. Firstly, because I didn't want to touch it. Secondly, because I was worried that making contact with it would compromise its sterility. Something I'm sure you straights are too busy to think of while you're actually doing the "dirty" deed.

Janis sat up. "Did David leave?"

"I think he's on his way out."

"Well, get him to do another one!"

"Can they do it again?"

"He says he can!"

"David, wait! We need another one!"

From downstairs I heard a somewhat panicked "What?!," but he came through for us. What a good sport.

After a few more months of inseminating three times per cycle, Janis was late for her period. Since she was usually extremely regular, we became excited. A week went by, then eight days, nine. Janis's breasts were swollen. She felt very premenstrual. She was snippy and moody. She had all the signs!

We were visiting some pals, and we just had to share what we hoped was "the news." Janis couldn't help but become weepy and flushed: two more indicators of pregnancy! She went to the bathroom to wash her hot face. She came back ashen. She'd got her period. It was unusually heavy and painful. Our friends looked away, embarrassed by our naked sadness. Had Janis just lost the very beginnings of what might have been our baby?

We kept trying. At first, every month that it didn't take was a mini-grieving. After a while, Janis just put her shoulder down and kept at it. At some point, a well-meaning friend tried to commiserate by saying that Janis must feel like she was suffering a tragedy. Janis's response to me was, "I've been to slums in Delhi, seen oppression in Guatemala, and worked with street kids in Toronto. *This* is not suffering. This is not tragedy. This, we will get through one way or another."

I was still sickened by the roller-coaster ride of hope and despair each month. Slowly, I began to follow her lead.

IT'S STILL NOT WORKING

By the time we'd been at it for a year, the little cup of stuff and what we did with the syringe became completely unrelated to the idea of having a baby. It developed into a scheduling dance of three busy people's PalmPilots. We had almost no expectation of a result.

Part of our problem was probably age. We started trying when we were close to thirty-five. Some people imply that women should be punished for waiting too long, for trying to have it all: career, relationships, and children. Of course, Larry King can have kids in his sixties, and we're all supposed to be not icked out.

Some of my friends who started trying in their thirties also had trouble. Ellie is in the middle of it as I write this. She's an incisive, dimpled, lanky actor and comedian who co-starred with me in our brave but ill-fated sitcom. She finally admits that in some ways, she wishes she could use our method.

"I have peed on sticks at $50 a pop. I've slathered spit on Petri dishes, I've spindled my vaginal mucus. I now call pregnancy tests my $20 period starter. I think my womb is inhospitable – that doesn't shock anyone I say that to . . . weird. Quite frankly, the idea of a turkey baster seems much more practical and appealing – I don't want my guy's penis getting in my way. Just give me the sperm and I'll do it myself, for God's sake. Do I sound romantic?" – Ellie

After a year and a half of trying, we knew we'd hit a wall. We either had to go to a more invasive medical route, adopt, or . . . go to curtain number three: me.

PUSHING THE CAR

Janis broached the subject in typical unblinking fashion. She believed it was time I tried, and that I should just buck up and accept it. Up until then, I had considered myself more of a cheerleader, someone who was there to boost Janis's spirits. I never imagined it would take for me because I wasn't the mothering type. I was too small, busy, goofy. After all, I dress like a teenage boy. I talk baby-talk when I'm nervous. I still don't own a hutch. I can't cook. My CDs are in a holder made up of other CDs. I leave funny outgoing messages on my answering machine. I have an answering machine. There is a very dormlike aura about me that resists any attempts of conversion into domestic pulchritude.

But in the face of Janis's fierce confidence in me, and our combined "failure fatigue," I relented. I thought of it as helping her to push the car. So I blindly joined in. Expecting not to be expecting.

The logistics were daunting. Mostly, we split the syringe.

Janis was adamant that we should *both* try each month. Double our chances. Because I am Jewish and dramatic, I immediately assumed that the worst would happen. We'd both get pregnant at the same time! Who would rub *my* feet?!

We'd heard a story about friends-of-friends who inseminated at the same time and both got pregnant. With twins. All boys! Now, granted, these could be the same "friends-of-friends" who went to Mexico and brought back a dog that they later discovered was a rat. Or who had a huge bug bite and when it popped, baby spiders came out. Still, I allowed the two-twins story to freak me out.

My apocryphal hand-wringing did not dissuade Janis. So, if we were ovulating around the same time, I'd inseminate her, and she'd put the dregs in me. Or, if we weren't in synch, then David would have to come (sorry) to our house six times, sometimes within a few days, to give sperm for each of us. He joked that, in a Pavlovian response, every time he drove by our house, he got an erection.

The first time, as Janis neared me with the syringe, I shouted, "I'm backing out! I'm backing out!" kicking my feet at her to keep her at bay. Luckily, she persisted, and has a really strong grip.

Like any animal that's been bested, I submitted with a passive-aggressive sigh. I lay there limply with my knees in the air. Suddenly

I had a very bad feeling. I was sharply reminded that I had had a big jug of Gatorade to drink just before I got into position. Here I was with my legs in the air, butt up, having to pee so bad I felt sick.

"Sweetie, I'm sorry, but I have to get up and go pee," I said.

"No! You have to lie like that for twenty minutes or it won't take!"

"I'm peeeeing!" I ran to the bathroom and flushed our first month's efforts down the toilet.

Was I unconsciously sabotaging this procedure? Perhaps. The next month, my second cycle, we did it a bit late. I was past ovulating. I forgot to take my folic acid, and I was doing a play so I was up late at night, drinking with the gals in the cast. I figured there was just no way it'd take, so I kept on living what I thought was my life.

WHAT UP WITH *THAT*?!

I was performing in an all-female version of Shakespeare's *A Midsummer Night's Dream* when Janis and I first started inseminating at the same time. I was playing the powerful Fairy Queen, Titania, and the verbose King of Thebes, Theseus.

One night after a show I drank quite a lot of red wine and bummed cigarette after cigarette from a castmate, Waneta, as we shared theatre gossip: "I know, I can't believe she took him back, he's such an addict – pass me my wine."

The odd thing was that no matter how much I drank, I couldn't get a buzz on. I mused that I must be about to get my period. But wasn't it a week early?

After the show closed, Janis and I went to our little cabin in the bush three hours north of Toronto. It was early December and chilly with a blush of snow. We had just bought what had formerly been a hunt camp, and the evidence of middle-aged, arrested-development Bambi-killers was everywhere. Retro-porn playing cards were strewn about the cabin. A gallows for carcasses of deer hung behind it. Dozens of old beer and Pepsi cans were strewn among the trilliums. A half-burnt mattress was evidence of the former owner's decision to set fire to his furniture instead of bothering to carry it out.

We had our work cut out for us in making this place habitable, and exorcising it of its dirty, yokel, Elmer Fudd energy. We took on our new project with gusto.

Immediately, we realized we needed to build a new outhouse. The one used by the hunters was a write-off. Two words: *beer* and *aim*.

I am aware that as an urban Jew, I'm letting my brothers and sisters down by even going near a structure without indoor plumbing. However, like many women, my sense of identity was dependent upon who I was with at any moment. So, since my girl was into it, I was into it.

In order to build a new outhouse, we first had to dig a deep hole. I set to work digging. When Janis checked in with me, I was standing four feet into semi-frozen earth. I had done it all myself. She was stunned. Where did this Wonder Woman burst of strength and indefatigable energy come from?

A few nights later, Janis and I both got our periods – which ruined our romantic weekend. We were long past the stage of mourning the loss of a fertilized ovum so we didn't think much more of it. Then my period suddenly stopped. I had had a bit of light red blood, nothing else. And yet my breasts were sore and I felt really premenstrual. I was so sure that I wasn't pregnant that I drank red wine and smoked some pure Northern Ontario reefer. I had stopped taking folic acid, and I'm sure I ate shellfish – with a splash of unpasteurized cheese.

TESTING THE WATERS

By the time we got home, we started to get suspicious of what my earlier period had been. So we took our "dirty-till-it-hurts" selves to the local drugstore. I was convinced that the pregnancy test would simply be a mildly disappointing ritual on the way to a long bath.

As soon as we got home and took the stick out of the box, we became shaky. You have to pee on it and then let it sit for two minutes. If you are pregnant, you'll see two red lines. If not, you'll only have one. We promised each other that I'd pee, and we'd both leave the bathroom *without peeking at the lines.*

I held the stick between my legs and aimed it at my stream. I watched it to make sure it was getting enough pee on it. I had read that it needed ten seconds, and I wanted to do everything by the book. In looking down, I could already see a second red line starting to form. I looked away quickly, and pressed the image from my mind.

I capped the stick and put it on the flat surface of our bathroom shelves. Janis and I left and closed the door behind us. Offering the pee stick some privacy. I paced. Janis sat motionless in the hallway. One hundred and twenty seconds later we went back in.

Two. Red. Lines.

"Oh my my God oh my God oh my God oh my God." I sunk down onto the toilet seat, trembling and crying. Janis sat at my feet smiling insanely. She confessed that she had looked at the stick as I put it down and had seen the lines. I confessed that I had seen them as I peed. Our lives together as mothers had begun in boisterous deceit.

"This is big," I whispered.

Yes. It's the whole world.

A tip: Once you know when you're ovulating, experts suggest you try to conceive on that day, the next day, and two days later. Of course, some of you will just be doing it all the time. Many people I spoke with shared the titillating detail that the idea that sex was actually making a baby contributed to a super-human dose of horniness. That's a delightful bonus. Just don't creep your child out by telling them.

2

The First Weeks

I'm Backing Out!

Perhaps it's due to an overactive imagination, but I'm one of those people who hasn't felt the need to try new things.

We cried ourselves out and then contemplated what to do. We needed to call our donor daddy. We debated calling our parents. My well of emotion was met by Janis's sober contemplation.

"I can't believe you did it so *fast.*" She shook her head.

As if *I* had anything to do with it.

She wanted to wait to tell anyone until I could get to the doctor and get blood tests. I needed to tell someone right away.

I called David. He answered the phone and asked how up north was. I interrupted, "It's going to be a Jew baby." He took a minute to register what that meant. He whooped. He wept. He asked to speak to Janis. She swallowed her tears before she took the phone.

I suddenly realized what Janis had sacrificed by asking me to try to conceive instead of more aggressively pursuing her own fertility: her biological relationship to the child. And, as we would discover, legal rights and her standing in some people's eyes.

24

In that moment, we were bursting with joy and expectation. And very tender with each other. I decided to call a few more people.

Before I tackled my family, I called my oldest and best friend, Ruth, an actor and writer with the breezy comic everywoman appeal of a Jimmy Stewart. Ruth enjoys forcing us to go out for ice cream, but she makes me tell her that she's not fat first. She's 110 pounds. (When I told her that I'd be describing her this way in this book, she asked if I could say that she's 108 pounds.) She is my touchstone.

"Ruth, sit down, I have to tell you some news –," I began.

"Janis is pregnant!" she yelled.

"No. I am."

"Huh?"

Because I'd only been at it for two months and we'd had so many disappointments, I hadn't told her that I'd started trying. She kept repeating "Diane is pregnant" with the emphasis on a different syllable each time:

"*Diane* is pregnant."

"Diane *is* pregnant."

"Diane is *pregnant*?!"

Her husband said he wished he didn't know because he's superstitious. So he told me that he was happy for us and, "Now I'm going to pretend I don't know until, all's well, three months have passed."

Then and there I adopted the habit of compulsively saying "all's well" prior to any pronouncements about the future. This is a habit of my Jewish family, and it linked me with all sorts of other paranoid people – from Jewish and other neurotic cultures – around the world.

All this time Janis hadn't said much. She was looking up midwifery clinics on the Internet.

Next I called my sister, Laura. She lives in deepest, darkest middle America – Missouri – with her husband, Todd. Because she is both decisive and a hippie, she said that she felt that it was perfectly and cosmicly right that I get pregnant right away, and assured me that she would too. "I just know it will be the same for us when we start trying, which will probably be next year."

"All's well," I added.

She advised me that the folks would be so thrilled they'd be in danger of coronaries.

I called my mom, Lily. Fearing for her big, warm heart, I told her to sit. As kids we referred to mom as a "health nut." She'd had us on whole grains and organic meats long before it was fashionable. She's into Reiki and homeopathy, and never fails to e-mail us about the latest discoveries of toxins lurking in innocent materials like lipstick. A devoted and spectacular mother herself, I assumed she'd go bananas.

Her response was uncharacteristically underwhelmed for a joyful person who is generally unencumbered by subtlety, filters, or boundaries. "Well, that's amazing. I didn't know you were trying. Isn't that wonderful? Does David know yet? You'll have to get a naturopath. My homeopath is right near you. Well, of course I wish you all the best."

She unceremoniously handed the phone to my father, Cy. His voice was soft, "That's great news. I didn't know you were trying. *Mazel tov*, Dolly."

I hung up, upset. A grandchild is something they'd been yearning for. They love me. They love Janis. What was this? Maybe they really are being hit in the face with this lesbian thing. Maybe they've actually disapproved of us having children this whole time.

This would not be an uncommon reaction. A lesbian couple that we met recently had a more concise response from a relative.

"My aunt calls herself a Christian, what she said was along the lines of 'Your child will be a bastard. What you're doing is against God.' But, when that little baby came, the tune was instantly changed to 'What a sweet little lucky baby you are to have two mommies to love you.' – Lorna

Lorna got whiplash from her aunt's sudden change of heart, but a real live baby can work miracles.

I called my older brother, Dan. He's a sweet soul who loves kids and is my biggest fan and supporter. His response was total glee. He erupted in high-pitched peels of laughter. I took this moment to get serious with him, something we don't do very often. "You will make a great uncle and that child will be so lucky to have you to – oh, other line, maybe it's Mom calling back – gotta go, bye."

"Okay, tell me the whole thing again from the beginning," she gulped into the phone.

"Are you happy?" I was aware that no one can hurt me like her.

"I was shocked. I'm starting to get bubbles. It's a wonderful thing!"

Laura called back on the other line. I told her mom was all right. I clicked back to my mother, who was now *mazel tov*-ing and all's well-ing and wanting to talk to Janis, offering all help and love, and planning planning planning. I got off the phone, exhausted. I offered it to Janis. She still didn't want to call anyone. She wanted to be quiet and ponder. We didn't know what to do now. Go out for dinner? Discuss our parenting philosophies? Make love? Make lists?

Within the next week, we headed to Janis's parents for Christmas brunch. Janis and her family are on the other end of the expressiveness continuum from my family. Their roots are good Canadian/British WASP. They are very loving, kind, and generous. Quietly so. Janis's two siblings, a brother and a sister, are also gay.

We went to pick up Janis's brother, Ian, from a Starbucks in the heart of Toronto's gay village. As usual, he looked flawless, in pressed Levi's, a fitted dark sweater, and a faux leather jacket.

He strolled to our car and folded his long legs into our cramped back seat. In his hands were two lattes, one of which he offered to me. The smell of my formerly most favourite breakfast food revolted me. I got hit by a wave of nausea.

Janis told him our news. He was thrilled in a typically under-stated way — he smiled, his face got red, and he squeezed my arm. Then he spent the car ride telling us how, if men could have babies, he never would. You couldn't pay him enough money to do it. "You're very brave," he told me gravely. As a medical researcher, he had lots of information about what I was about to go through. "Not for a million dollars," he repeated.

He promised that he would teach the kid the most important thing about life: style. Janis said that it was perfect that I was preg-nant because I love babies, and she loves kids. "And I love cats," Ian added, looking out the back window. Then he detailed facts for us about nausea and boob pain. "Well, that's how it was in *my* first trimester," he deferred.

At her parents' condominium, I waited for Janis to break the news. I knew it was her call. Yet, I was surprised by her compo-sure. I was sweating (and burping — more on that later).

After an hour or so, we sat at the table. Janis was looking at Christmas cards and there was one with a picture of a newborn on it. She held it out to her mom, Doris, and said, "Oh, we have news."

Doris looked at Janis and said, "Which one?" Janis pointed to me. Doris smiled and her whole face was pink. She said, "Isn't that great, and, well, wonderful news." Then, after a classic comedy beat, she turned back to Janis and cracked us all up with a zinger, "What's wrong with *you*?"

Janis's dad reminded us that it was a bit early still and we had to be careful. "But most of these things turn out all right." His version of "all's well."

That night we had Hanukkah dinner at my parents. My brother,

Dan, gave me the first of many presents he was to buy for us, the book *Chicken Soup for the Expectant Mother's Soul*. (I knew I was really pregnant a few nights later when, instead of curling my toes and making cynical comments about the mass-market, emotionally manipulative pap that I thought the *Chicken Soup* stuff was, I sat there with tears rolling down my cheeks, whacking Janis on the arm every few minutes to show her another chapter. "'My Father's Tears.' Isn't that beautiful?")

Also at Hanukkah dinner was Janis's oldest and best friend, Netty. Netty's an outdoor adventure enthusiast whose day job is to work with the hardest-to-house schizophrenic street people. She's the person you want with you when you're in an elevator and someone creepy walks on.

When we told her, Netty's eyes shone with tears. She knew intimately how long we had hoped for this – since Janis tells her everything. She hugged us firmly, and said loudly (for this is the only way Netty can speak) over and over to me, "I just can't believe you!"

That night, I joked about getting fat, and later at home I danced around with sore boobs, singing that I'd still be sexy with a big ass and belly. We were hanging in a cloud of bliss. Little nausea, no pain, just the promise of a dream.

RESPONSES TO REMEMBER
People seem to love warning you of dire things the moment they find out you've got a bun in there:

> "Well, you better be careful. You're already fat." – Netty's mother

> "When I was about thirteen or fourteen weeks' pregnant, a friend's mother said that she was happy for me but that I could still lose the baby." – Laura

"No sugar, no carbs, honey." – Ramona's mom

"Your life, as you know it, is over." – A grocery-store clerk, to me

You never really know how your news will affect someone. Although you expect tears of joy and congratulations, you can't know what someone else might be dealing with.

A friend of my sister's had suffered a miscarriage the year before. The first time she saw Laura pregnant, "She looked at me with intensity in her eyes and said in a low guttural voice, 'I want that. . . .'"

At the time that I got pregnant, a friend of mine was going through a tremendous loss. So although it was really early, I told her our news. I hoped the promise of new life might lift some of her sadness. That the insanity that it was me – goofy, old, pratfalling me – who got pregnant might make her laugh. When I told her, she squatted down into a monkey position with legs wide open, bounced up and down over and over, laughing and bellowing, "It's gonna *hurt*! It's gonna *hurt*!" We both cracked up. However, she also introduced me to the term *ring of fire*.

Another good buddy of mine, who had been trying to get pregnant as long as Janis had, said that she was not surprised. "You just stick your finger in the water and boom. You know how to do it."

Even though I was not sure what she meant, I thought it was sweet. I didn't suspect that there might be sadness behind her congratulations. I was already losing my perspective and sensitivity to others. My growing fecundity was taking over.

SECOND THOUGHTS – THE FIRST FEW WEEKS
Perhaps it's due to an overactive imagination, but I'm not one of those people who feels the need to try new things. I scare easily. I

could never coax myself to ingest hallucinogens, even when my friend Shael told me that while on acid, he'd seen Jesus. Apparently Christ quoted all the words to the song "Blinded by the Light" by Bruce Springsteen (clearing up that controversy about the lyric "wrapped up like a douche another roamer in the night"). At amusement parks, I was the kid holding the other kids' cotton candy while they rode roller coasters. Skydiving, singing karaoke, and eating frogs' legs are not activities I'll be trying before I die.

So after I got pregnant I focused on getting informed and prepared. I read all sorts of pregnancy books in the hopes that the knowledge I found would calm any fears I had. (Please see the reference section in the back of this book for some suggestions.) Many of the books served to agitate me further, especially when they talked breezily of pain, loss of ambition, the fact that you might not ever get your body back.

The night I completed my read-a-thon was Janis and my seventh anniversary. After dinner, I broke down and told her some of my fears. "This will change our whole life," I sniffled as I clung to her. "Will we ever be able to snuggle together and watch a video again? Is this an idea I adopted like a new puppy and will want to give back to the Humane Society? Are we doing this because other people are doing it? Will you love me when my boobs look like rocks in socks?! I'm backing out!"

Janis reminded me of something our friend Patricia, a Medusa-haired, successful, and irreverent filmmaker (and mother of two) told us years earlier:

"When I got pregnant, many of my friends, family, and complete strangers felt it necessary to shake their heads, look at my belly, and say, 'Yer life's gonna change now, you know.' I would shrug and say, 'And what made you think I wanted it to stay the same?'"

"Besides," Janis added, "who has ever regretted having a child?" I wondered silently to myself: Me?

Janis said honestly that sometimes she wondered why after trying for so long, the pregnancy didn't take for her. "I was up at bat for a year, and you hit a home run on the first try." I couldn't say why, and I didn't want her to feel like she'd failed at something that has to do with nothing but fate, but she knew this already, so I just told her how much I loved her.

Happy anniversary.

FIRST SYMPTOMS:
SIGNS OF TOTAL AND COMPLETE CHANGE

A few days later, I started to gag. I wasn't really nauseous, just gaggy. It was kind of exciting. The heave-reflex happened and I threw my arms out as if to say, "Cool, huh?"

One morning Janis had her head on my chest and her leg up and across me, and I unconsciously had my right hand extended as a barrier to her getting her heavy knee anywhere near my queasy stomach.

She was cuddling me when suddenly I had the urge to barf. I tried to untangle myself from her – to roll away and lean my head over the side of the bed. She thought I was playing friskily and clung to me. It became a slightly comical struggle, until I finally broke free and bucked with dry heaves. As she realized what happened, she felt terribly guilty. "I didn't know you were sick. You were acting like *you*."

I didn't want not to be *me* either, so I made a joke of it. "I'm still *me*, I'm just disgusting."

A few days later, Janis and I went for a run. I felt pretty confident I could handle her usual seven-kilometre route. I was only six weeks' pregnant at this point.

A cousin of David's told us that she ran a marathon when she was six weeks' pregnant. No problem. Well, she did end up getting pneumonia and had to be hospitalized for weeks, "but really," she assured us, her tight blouse and jeans hugging her taught seven-month-pregnant body, "pregnancy doesn't have to be a drag."

I could barely make it up the hill near the end of our run. I was beyond slow. My limbs were molten rubber. I couldn't seem to breathe properly. I became irritated. I was reminded that I hate jogging. What a stupid sport. Running for no reason like a moron. Nobody's chasing us, are they? How often in life are you called upon to *run*? I might as well be doing trigonometry!

I was, however, secretly disappointed with myself. I didn't want to be giving up my newly toned-and-trim body this soon. Yet, I could feel that things were irrevocably changing.

Both my parents seemed to want me to carry on as before. My mother assured me that although she threw up every day on the hour for nine months, she still worked throughout her first trimester, in the snow, without shoes.

My father asked what else was going on. When I replied, "Who cares?" he pushed delicately to see if I had any acting or writing work coming up.

I did care of course, but I was less panicked about work. What a gift that was! For the first time in my career, I wasn't constantly beating the bushes for the next possibility. And strangely, work came to me. I found myself busier with writing projects than I had been in a long while.

Moreover, we already had a part-time job. Pregnancy. We took on this "project" like the thirty-something, urban professionals we are. We got on the Net. We looked up midwives versus obstetricians.

MIDWIVES VERSUS OBGYNS

Janis and I discovered that in Ontario, you can either have a midwife or an OBGYN, not both. Being on record as feminists, we were keen to check out what midwives could offer. A woman-centred medical service outside of the mainstream world of big bucks and bigger egos appealed to our "personal-is-political" mindsets. We knew that globally, midwives have been delivering babies for thousands of years. We understood that it's only in the last hundred or so that the medical establishment, sensing the plus-sized profits that babies being born every day could reap, pathologized and co-opted childbirth.

But I am still a middle-class girl with an overactive sense of doom, so I wanted to make sure that we could deliver the baby in the hospital, surrounded by all the technology available to assist the new one (all's well, should anything happen, which of course it wouldn't, God forbid, but you never know, better to be prepared, just in case) in its first moments out on the town.

Ruth recommended her OB to us. One of the best in the city. Ruth told us that the appointments were once a month and didn't start until you were past your first trimester. The appointments lasted about fifteen minutes each, which didn't sound like much time to me. Ruth worried that midwives might be too airy-fairy, not up to speed with the latest techniques. I'm sure she imagined them sitting cross-legged in a nest of non-bleached cotton pillows on an unsterilized clay floor, hair tangled to their waists, entoning together as they breathed in the spirits of women's suffering and breathed out the patriarchy.

We went to interview midwife clinics. They would meet with us immediately, unlike the OBs. Many of my theatre friends recommended a clinic called The Midwife Collective. We arrived in a bright, cheery medical office full of baby pictures. The receptionist, Jocelyn, had an earring in her eyebrow and an angelic smile. The senior midwife, Joyce, took us into her office. Although there *was* a futon, there was also a computer.

Joyce is a genial, salt-and-pepper-haired pro. A mother herself, she'd been at this long before it was covered by OHIP. She told us that your midwife can order all the same tests as your doctor would – ultrasounds, genetic screening, blood tests – and they spend an hour per appointment with you, not a cursory fifteen minutes. In Toronto, midwives have privileges at the major hospitals, so I could have my birth there, and if there were any problems, they'd call in the attending OBs. After any interventions by hospital staff, care would be transferred back to the midwife, who would be with us from the beginning until the bitter end.

After the birth, midwives would come to us on the first day, and three more times in the first week. They'd continue postnatal care for six weeks. Not only did they offer comprehensive personal care, but their emphasis was on maternal involvement and "choice." We nodded our heads earnestly as Joyce told us how important it was for a woman to have some say in her pregnancy and birth. Not to be steamrolled by a medical system that has money and time as its greatest pressures.

As she talked about hospitals' rates of C-sections and episiotomies, birth plans and home births, the list of tests we could choose to undergo and the ones that were medically imperative, I found myself zoning out. The room was warm. The sound of Joyce's gentle voice lulled me into a honey-dipped haze. . . . Honey-dipped equals doughnut. Doughnuts equal grease. Grease equals smelly equals barf! I gagged. Joyce stopped and registered where I was at. "Oh, you've got it bad already. Well, there is a very safe drug we can prescribe if you choose."

I loved her immediately.

As we walked the hallway and scanned the corkboards filled with baby pictures, Joyce told us that if a pregnancy becomes high risk – if there are twins or if the mother develops gestational diabetes or high blood pressure – she is transferred to an OB for the rest of her pregnancy. Midwives can handle most things in the range of a normal pregnancy. Positive that I would not develop anything beyond "the norm," we chose The Midwife Collective.

When we got home, I called my mother to tell her of our decision. My mother is stupendously informed about a staggering range of topics. She works for herself as an academic counsellor, rescuing kids that are struggling in school. She also has a part-time job: worrying.

"How are you?" she asked, her tone descending as if talking to someone whose answer would be "Dying."

"Tired," I responded. "But good," I added excitedly, so she wouldn't worry.

It didn't work.

"Tired? Something must be wrong. You should see a naturopath."

I told her that I was going to see a midwife. I thought she'd be reassured by this news.

She asked, "A naturopathic midwife?"

I didn't know if there was any such thing, but my thought was, Isn't a midwife cool enough?!

A call came through on the other line, freeing me to struggle with my complex feelings about my mother another time.

It was cute Jocelyn with the pierced eyebrow and the neck tattoo from The Midwife Collective. They had made an appointment to see me again at week ten, not twelve. That was important. I was starting to feel very, very sick.

— • • • —

A tip on telling: Some cultures have a tradition of waiting to tell the news until the end of the first trimester, in case of miscarriage. Most women whom I spoke with who'd endured a miscarriage mentioned that the silence around it made it that much harder to overcome. My suggestion about spilling the beans would be, before twelve weeks, tell those people who you'd normally turn to for good or bad news.

— • • • —

3

The First Trimester

Losing Control

You get the feeling that some other primal part of you is driving your body, and you're not even in the back seat, you're in the trunk . . . and you're running out of air.

To say that my first trimester was consuming would be an understatement. Everything was stark and foreign. As a result, sensations, emotions, and revelations were experienced to their fullest. They were dissected by and discussed with the most unsuspecting friends, family, and telemarketers.

Looking back on it now, I feel so desperately lucky. How often as adults do we embark on the adventure of doing something truly for the first time? In those instances, good or bad, we really live in the moment. It's a rich and innocent state.

Even if it is accompanied by the sensitivity to smell, the moods, the brain shrinkage, the disgusting nausea and vomiting, the exhaustion, the weepiness, the body-changing weight gain, the g-a-s, the thrill, the panic, the rethinking of your whole focus and identity, the terror of "am I like my mother," the whole shebang.

MORNING SICKNESS AND OTHER ENCHANTING SYMPTOMS

Have I mentioned that one of my greatest fears (besides bugs frolicking in my ear canal and being trapped with a windbag at a party) is vomiting? So when I got pregnant I talked to everyone I knew about morning sickness.

"I only threw up once, when I brushed my tongue." – Zoe, mother of one

Anyone who would brush her tongue under any circumstances, much less in the grip of morning sickness, should expect to vomit.

"I was nauseous much of the time, but I dealt with it by eating as soon as the nausea came on and taking lots of naps, and I never actually threw up." – Ruth, mother of two

Ruth is sort of perfect. Her eating-all-the-time strategy appealed to me.

"My first trimester was a bliss time full of yummy hormones, and all I wanted to do was lie in a field of flowers and have gnomes tell me stories." – Wendel, mother of one

Sounded good.

Yet, many of the books I read told of women who interrupted presentations at board meetings to go throw up in trash cans, women who threw up on the bus, in restaurants, in class. The impression I got was that these women were like soldiers who hacked off their hanging, shrapnelled limbs and got back out there into the world without complaint. Well, I complained. Because I did not have a mild tongue-brushing case of morning sickness. Or even a case of "morning" sickness. I threw up all day, every day, into the night.

EXTREME SPORTS

It's been said about the first trimester that this is the time you *really* need that seat on the bus, but no one's going to give it to you.

Although the symptoms may be most intense during this time, you won't be showing yet, and often might not be telling anyone that you're pregnant. To cover up my constant absences from events and my dismaying countenance, we resorted to saying that I had stomach flu. For eighteen weeks.

A sporty, young musician friend of ours, Lisa, came by to visit a few times during what she had no idea was my first trimester. If I came down to say hi at all, she saw a grey-green puddle in sweatpants, with a greasy ponytail, drag itself halfway down the stairs, grunt and half-smile in recognition, and slowly ooze back up to bed. The third time Lisa popped by I overheard her telling Janis, "Wow, Diane's really had a lot of stomach flus this winter. Maybe she's carrying a parasite."

"Maybe," smiled Janis, "maybe."

I have no idea why an extreme version of first trimester symptoms happened to me. I was told that I had a high level of maternal hormones. The midwives said that a high hormonal level and intense symptoms were a good thing. Yes, there was a positive spin to be put on this. It meant the pregnancy would probably "take" and there was less chance of miscarriage. Or it could mean I was carrying twins. Or it could mean I was simply unlucky.

Odette, a colleague of Janis's, had severe vomiting like mine. We clung to each other, milking each other's stories of misery and triumph. She barfed for eighteen weeks. She took a medication that was later prescribed to me, Diclectin (a mix of vitamin B6 and antihistamine) and assured me that it was fine and safe.

In an e-mail, she recounted how she couldn't do any housework, even though she had to take time off work, and how that affected her relationship with her husband.

"He'd come home from work to find dirty dishes piled to the sky in the kitchen because I just could not face the smell. I would cry in the bathroom because it began to hurt my throat every time I threw up. I had very morbid thoughts. (I tell you, major hormonal swings.) I do not think I will eat another Premium Plus soda cracker ever in my life. But I would do it all over again." – Odette, mother of two

With Odette's second pregnancy she was sick once more, and this time, it lasted for the whole nine and a half months. Near the end of her term, she had to be hospitalized for dehydration. She recently told us that she had decided to stop at two kids.

Another friend, Mina, refused to take any medication. She just toughed it out and still got to work each day. Well, Odette and I smirked, *she* only threw up in the mornings. Amateur.

"My wife threw up on me on the train as we were commuting to work. She started to cry because she was so embarrassed. I said, 'Honey, don't cry. I'm the one with vomit all over my shirt.'" – Paul, father of two

Charlotte Brontë managed to survive the consumption (tuberculosis) that killed each of her siblings in turn. Maria and Elizabeth in 1825, Branwell and Anne in 1849, and Emily in 1848. But Charlotte died in 1855 of *hyperemesis gravidarum*, excessive vomiting during pregnancy, just three weeks shy of her thirty-ninth birthday.

Odette and I feel terribly lucky to live in this century when instead of actually dying from morning sickness, we just *wanted* to die.

TOO POOPED TO PUKE

"I felt like I woke up every morning with a hangover – without the benefit of having been drunk." – Tammy, composer, mother, and former workaholic

Besides the nausea, the symptom that knocks most women flat on their bodacious booties is intense exhaustion. Mind-numbing, body-dragging, bone-tired sleepiness. It's like having a low-grade fever, complete with chills and shakes, for three months.

My exhaustion was so thick that I felt like I was in a constant fog. What I could make out of the world was muffled by the sound of my own hormone-thickened blood slushing in my ears. My body became a dense, hungry, angry animal that took control of my being. So, any thinking, reasonable, good-humoured part of my mind was left to wander dark and drafty mental hallways with nothing but a tiny candle to light its way to nowhere.

Of course, some women I spoke to just felt a little pooped by dinnertime. But we don't talk to them any more.

I once overheard Janis telling someone that when she came home from work she would expect to find me in one of three positions: lying on the couch with a barf bucket beside my head; lying in bed with a barf bucket beside my head; face down on the bathroom floor.

The most trying way that this affected our relationship was that I felt like I was absent. I was not driving the car formally known as "me." I wasn't even in the backseat. I was in the trunk. And running out of air.

BURPING, FARTING, AND SPITTING – AH, THE GLAMOUR

In many cases the sickness of the first trimester starts slowly, almost sneakily. At my seventh week, I still had a sense of humour about it.

One day Janis was making a list of things to do around the house, with items like "paint shelves, go for a run at 4:00, phone Aunty Mary" – so I made a list too:

• burp
• gag
• gag
• fart
• spit
• burp
• gag
• burp

I managed to get through it pretty well.

In the first trimester, there is a lot of gas. People will warn you about this politely, but if you're standing too close, a pregnant woman's morning belch could blind you. And there's no point in a pregnant woman trying to stifle her burps, she'll give herself a hernia. Moms-to-be can shame most frat boys. "Belching the alphabet, fellas? No problem. Can you recite the value of Pi?" Speaking of "frat," the gas rumbles about in your lower GI as well.

When I was about nine weeks' pregnant, I was invited to join a writing workshop that met every Wednesday night for two hours. I didn't know how to tell the instructor that I was reluctant to attend because it was hard to sit in a room full of strangers for two hours without farting. Especially at night, which is prime farting time. I ended up going and taking frequent (and less and less discreet) breaks for "air."

I also had a lovely symptom that I haven't heard too many other women describe. Constant spitting. Some women experience an increase in saliva, or a different taste and consistency of their saliva. In my case, slobber would pool in my mouth and I'd have to spit it out to get rid of it. When I got too tired, I'd just let it run out of my slack jaw into a napkin, or after a long day, my shirt. By the end of the day I'd have a drool rash, just like a teething infant's. This bizarre symptom would disappear as quickly as it came. Each morning I'd wake up and hold my breath – would it be a saliva-free day or another twenty-four hours of yearning for a spittoon? On the spit days, I'd end up shutting myself in the house, lest random people think I was a) lusting after them or b) disgusting. I have no idea how my partner still managed not to be repulsed – or not to tell me about it.

WHAT STINKS?!

Yes, the smells! It's true. A woman's sense of smell increases to dog-like sensitivity when she's pregnant. They say that this is to protect you from ingesting anything that might harm your baby like tobacco, alcohol, unpasteurized cheeses, kitty litter, or KFC. I wanted to wear a cape with a big nose on it, "Super Shnoz!" Unfortunately Super Shnoz can't always be trusted to know exactly what she's smelling.

At about twelve weeks along I attended a theatre community gathering. It was my first night out in a while. I was still pale and sick, but was happy to be among friends, and to be far enough along that we could start officially spreading the good news. I was standing beside an actor friend of mine, Richard, who is like a brother to me. A cute (he's fifty), slightly dishevelled, sticky-fingered brother. Suddenly I smelled pee. I was sure that someone must have literally pissed themselves. Well, who would be inadvertently walking around in stinky pee pants but Richard? I looked around in horror to the other people in the little circle I was chatting with. I thought, Dear God, we are standing in Richie's pee and everyone is too polite to say anything. Then I realized the smell of urine was coming from his beer. It took me a moment to understand. Beer smelled like pee to me. Just like wine smelled like someone left a vinegar bottle in a shoe.

I could smell Nutrasweet. Did you know it has a smell? It does and it smells like rust. Luckily Nutrasweet is bad for you, so I didn't mind giving it up. It becomes relatively easy for pregnant women to wean themselves off of drinking alcohol, being any-where near smoke, and drinking coffee. It's nature's little gift to puking mamas and their babies.

When my mother was pregnant in the mid-1960s, her doctor said that she *could* smoke. In fact, he suggested that it would help her not gain too much weight. (She was told that she wasn't sup-posed to put on more than twenty-five pounds.) She was also encouraged to keep drinking alcohol if it kept her calm. The doctor who recommended this also prescribed thalidomide during her barfy first trimester. (Luckily, she didn't take it since thalido-mide was later discovered to cause birth defects in some children.)

Besting addictions is a positive effect of the hormones. Losing your mental capacities is not.

HAS ANYONE SEEN MY HEAD?

We moms refer to it as "brain shrinkage." This occurs when you wash your hair with bubble bath and put your phone in the bra drawer.

Before I got pregnant I was pretty sharp. Some people thought I was quite a smart young woman, but now, not so much. During pregnancy, words escaped me. I had trouble with simple sentences like, "Honey, can you pass the uh . . . the . . . uh . . . the thingmajig . . . the yellow whachamacall . . . that goes on the bread?"

"Butter?"

"No, no, it smells like gasoline. The whosy."

"Margarine?"

"No! It's for the uh . . . the long stringy whadgacallit that kids eat?"

"Cheese?"

"No! In a bun . . . the whatsitsname in a bun –"

"Hot dog?"

"Thank you. Yes. And can you put the yellow sauce on it, not ketchup, but –"

"Mustard?"

"*Yes!*"

"We only have honey mustard."

"Oh, don't make me puke!"

The most shameful incident of loss of intellectual faculties involved our dog, a hairy, big-headed, Akita-shepherd cross named Stanley. One night around midnight I bolted awake from a sound sleep. I had a bad feeling. It was too still in the house, too empty. Something was wrong. I thought, The dog's being awfully quiet. Hope he's all right. I went downstairs to look for him, and he wasn't there. I looked outside. I started to panic. I opened the door and called him. No dog. I woke Janis up to ask her in halting sentences that brought on burps and gagging where the dog was.

"Maybe he's . . . braaap . . . lost . . . or . . . acckkk . . . run off?! Maybe he's jealous . . . pffffft . . . of the baby!" She reminded me that I had had the dog with me when I dropped off a video at the store before going to bed. "OH. MY. URRP. GOD." I ran outside in my pyjamas. I could just make out the silhouette of his huge head in the backseat of our car. He'd been sitting there for three hours.

Luckily it was a balmy night. I let him out of the car. He stretched, yawned, and gave me a lick. He wasn't even upset. This distressed me even more. I grabbed his big scruffy neck and burst into tears. Not knowing what else to do, I apologized profusely to him. His neck smelled like a dishrag, which smelled like the garbage can, which smelled like the river and the inside of an oven. I crouched in the middle of the street hugging Stanley, crying and retching by moonlight.

Janis tried to find some humour in what happened. I was inconsolable. How could I trust myself with a human baby?! Would I leave him/her in the car? How would our child survive the wreck that is me? Even Janis couldn't reassure me. All I could do was gnaw on my guilt and resolve to always, *always* check the back seat.

FIRST TRIMESTER MOODS – DUCK!

"If you have a few silly ideas come into your head, just put them out again and think of something pure, lovely and of good report. We all have silly ideas come into our heads sometimes, but they do no harm if we just think of something else, or go for a walk. Cheer up and be happy." – Helen MacMurchy, *The Canadian Mother's Book*, 1931

Hormones can change a loved one's personality so drastically, it may become unclear who they really are. Your formerly adorable angel may occasionally morph into a combination of Roseanne, Mister Hyde, and Blanche Dubois. The only consolation is that it is much more disconcerting to her than it is to you. The best thing you can do for her is to get past it. Or get out of the way.

My dear, mad-genius friend Bruce told me that, "Statistically, the rate for husbands murdering their wives increases when the wife is pregnant. It's a male animal flight response." He joked that when his wife, Tracey, was pregnant, he constantly reassured her that he was not going to kill her. What he doesn't know is that she just might have killed him.

A husband of a friend of mine took me aside one afternoon at a brunch. In hushed tones, he asked me how Janis was coping. I started to say how supportive and kind she was, how she put up with my loss of personality, capacities, and epiglottal control. He interrupted, "No, I mean how is she coping with your *moods*." I told him that the hormones were mostly making me spew, not snap. "Lucky her. I'm still recovering ten years later. I think a lot of those moods are in your head anyway."

I was so shocked by the last statement that I didn't ask him how it was that he could accept that hormones could do a little thing like create life from thin air, and provide the balanced food to support it, but if a mother gets a little testy it's "all in her head."

The dismissive mythology around women and our emotional states got really annoying to me when I was pregnant. So here's a news flash: *Mood swings in pregnancy are real, and while we're at it, so is PMS.* Let's all just accept each other's endocrine systems once and for all. I personally don't ever have the urge to go out and hit an inanimate object really hard with a stick, but I respect that some men are hormonally driven to do so. A pregnant woman is doing life's most important job, so let her get a little snippy.

Before I got pregnant, I was relatively easygoing, anyone could tell you that. But not any more. One crisp winter day, Janis and I were out for a drive. Janis was behind the wheel and I was in the passenger seat reading the newspaper. Janis kept taking quick, furtive glances at the headlines as she was driving. This is a cute habit Janis has had for years. Suddenly, I found it intensely irritating. As patiently and sweetly as I could, I said, "Honey, do you think you could stop reading the newspaper while you're driving, FER FUCK'S SAKE?!"

Those last three words exploded from my mouth. We both gasped. It was like someone had unzipped my skull and a foul-mouthed serpent came popping out wearing a fright wig. From then on, I tried desperately to remember to speak gently to Janis, who would spend the next nine months following me around, picking up the little pieces of my mind that had wandered off, like toddlers at the zoo. But it just didn't fly. I had no control:

"Do you think you could close the fridge door, fer fuck's sake?!"

"Could you please throw out that godawful, putrid, flowery incense, fer fuck's sake?"

"Could you not breathe like that? Like through your nose like that? Shh with the breathing, darling, fer fuck's frikkin flippin' sake!"

It came to a head one day when I was listening to my answering machine. Janis called out, "Pause it. Pause it."

I couldn't hear her, "What?" I mumbled. I was sitting there sick as a dog with my chin on my desk. Typing the word *blech* in all the different fonts. **blech** blech **blech**

"I want to listen to that!" Janis snapped.

"Okay." I slouched. And I just let the tape keep playing.

blech **blech** *blech*

"Stop the tape. Diane, I need to hear that. Why didn't you stop it?"

"Well, then rewind it and listen to it yourself, fer fuck's sake! Why are you yelling at me, fer fuck's sake?!" I slammed my desk repeatedly in frustration and glared at her.

Janis burst out laughing. I burst into tears. Janis held me as I sobbed unrelentingly. She reassured us both that it was about time I got in touch with my anger. "Good for you!" she even said. That was then.

In our relationship we always had a nifty balance. Janis had a short fuse, but got over anger fast. I had a longer fuse, but when I did get angry I stayed that way for a long time, i.e., I sulked. The balance worked for us. When "fer fuck's sake" started, my fuse was much shorter, and yet, I sulked longer. In order to keep our delicate homeostasis from swinging wildly out of whack, we had to make a game of my new-found temper. We ended every sentence with "fer fuck's sake" just for fun:

"Your mom called, fer fuck's sake."

"Buy some cheese, fer fuck's sake."

"That's a pretty blouse, fer fuck's sake."

Unfortunately, this all played havoc with my identity. Many women mentioned that the physical and emotional chaos of the first trimester tested their sense of their essential selves. It made them silently question the relationships closest to them. I remember feeling terribly disconnected from my partner, looking at her as if from a great height. Since my "no touch zone" started at my chin and wrapped itself around my body, her caress was painful and brought on waves of gagging. I no longer shared her sense of humour (or anyone's for that matter), I could do no physical activities with her. I fell asleep during most conversations. I didn't like anything or want anything. I was entirely self-involved.

During those times the words that kept repeating in my head were "I'm not up for this" and "I'm backing out!" I felt like I was being tested, and if I failed, I would be sure to be unmasked as a lousy person, partner, and mother. My true nature as a weak and spineless phony would be revealed. I believed that I couldn't cope with this, and if I couldn't handle this part, how would I handle labour? Or motherhood?

These dark thoughts contributed to a feeling of isolation, but it was at a dinner party one evening that I officially became a pariah. Not only could I not help but make an "ew-y" face and a barely audible "uchh" sound each time I picked a scallop out of my pasta and plunked it onto Janis's plate, but I spent the night glumly watching other people being hilarious and was not able to join in the laughter. All I could talk about was how no one talks about this feeling. This overwhelming feeling to talk about nothing else. I saw people's eyes glaze over in boredom and then horror when I repeatedly said things like, "Oh and the burping! No one mentioned that!" I knew they expected me to be overjoyed and thrilled and grounded in maternity. I couldn't. I was like a patient who was too overwhelmed by her illness to think of anything or anyone else.

When I got home, I was bleak, depressed, and couldn't stop crying. I just wanted to be alone, but was terrified of being abandoned. I wanted to talk of nothing but the baby, but was afraid of being trapped with it. I wanted people to know how debilitating this first trimester felt, but didn't want to be pathologized. I was a mess.

Yet all this psychic storm was manageable compared to what did me in, what I feared most, what made me lose track of the *point*

of all this sickness (the fact that a baby comes out in the end) —
the vomiting.

THE SKINNY ON THE SPEWING

Although it was all-day sickness, I didn't just lie there and take it.
I tried to combat it. Everyone I met seemed to have a cure. People
who have no frikkin clue what you are going through will
suggest some of the following coping mechanisms in the name of
being helpful:

- ginger
- ginger tea
- ginger ale (enough with the ginger already!)
- lemon juice
- vitamin B6
- almonds (for the vitamin B6)
- crackers
- acupuncture
- homeopathic remedies
- massage (don't touch me)
- exercise (I can't move)

One of the kitschier cures was wearing those seasickness bracelets that sailors use. The "bracelets" look like groovy 1970s tennis
sweatbands with a little red dot in the centre. The dot needs to be
positioned exactly three fingers from your wrist in the middle of
your forearm. It will hit a pressure point and trick your brain into
not feeling nauseous. Well, matie, it's not my brain that's barfing.

The most demoralizing upchucks were always when I would
throw up the remedies that other people suggested for the throwing up. I'd drink ginger tea and heave. I'd painstakingly and with
shaky hands squeeze the juice from six lemons, drink it, and

immediately regurgitate it into the sink. I'd try to hydrate in order to compensate for the water loss of constant retching so that I wouldn't die like a Brontë, and I'd end up instantly spitting up the water or juice or ginger ale until there was nothing left but the dry heaves. So I stopped drinking water, and then the crackers that I'd just eaten would gather in a clump and would sort of slide up my throat in slow motion and plop in a ball into the toilet. Which was preferable?

Another Catch-22–type gem occurred when I was barfing so much that I got the hiccups, and then the hiccups made me laugh, which made me barf.

Apparently, my mother's naturopathic dentist had a friend whose sister's cousin had terrible vomiting and all she did was take vitamin B6 and drink the juice of boiled barley grains and she was totally fine. In fact, she had tons of energy and started working out again! By the time I was told this suggestion, I was ready to throttle the next well-meaning soul who had a friend with a cure. The implication was that if I wasn't able to stop throwing up, something was wrong with *me*. It was all in my head, or I brought it on because of stress, or my attitude, or my karma, or my outfits.

In case someone judges you in this way, let me be clear: It is not your fault! Do not let anyone tell you that you should be feeling better and that if you're not it's because you are: too high-strung, too angry, too toxic, too negative, you're carrying a boy, you're carrying a girl, you don't really want your baby! Just know that it will pass and the result will be worth it.

You may even eventually find it funny. Looking back, some of the places that I threw up were pretty ridiculous:

- in the tub
- on the table by the bed
- in the bed

- in the elevator to the midwife's office
- behind a parked car
- while driving the car

One of my favourites occurred when Janis and I were walking Stanley through Cawthra Square Park. This half-acre of downtown Toronto park space is referred to as one of the most "colourful" parks in the city. It's inhabited by many homeless people, street kids, drug and alcohol users, dog walkers, cruising and/or strolling men and women, moms with kids, and the occasional jogger with a strong stomach. On a warm day, the plethora of smells can border on Eau de Dumpster.

Stanley, Janis, and I were almost through the park when big Stan stopped to do his business, and all of a sudden I had to stop too, to lean over and barf in the snow. Stanley seemed embarrassed by my behaviour and, in mid-poop, gave me a look as if to say, "Do you mind. I'm trying to void my bowels here." Then Janis gagged at the sight of me barfing, which made me barf some more. We were an excellent-looking family. The surrounding rubbies were seriously looking at making a complaint. I felt okay though, because everyone barfs in Cawthra Park.

Despite the festival of foulness, I consider myself lucky. I'm self-employed – also known as "often unemployed" – so I didn't have to show up to work. My sister, Laura, was sick at work and couldn't tell anyone for the first few weeks. She'd feel a gag coming on and lean over the garbage can by her desk in case she might vomit. One time she was leaning over, mouth open, when the dean of the department walked in. She pretended that she was looking for something she'd dropped. Her gum, maybe?

She'd also sneak out of business meetings early so she could go into the office of someone who was still in the meeting and sleep on their floor.

It is amazing how quickly we can adapt to a new reality. I began timing how fast I could feel a gag coming on, shuffle to the bathroom, drop to my knees, tie my hair in a scrunchy, take off my glasses, lift the toilet seat, barf, put the seat down, put on my glasses, and leave the bathroom. I got it down to a minute and a half. It's good multitasking practice for chasing after a toddler.

Many books will also tell you to make sure you take in certain foods and vitamins for your baby's nutritional needs, especially in the delicate first trimester. They will tell you this is your responsibility as a mother. They will imply that it's the least you can do to keep your baby alive. However, my midwife explained to me that your fetus is a self-centred little thing. It *will* get all the nutrients it needs from your body. *You* may end up anemic, pale, feeble, starving – with black circles under your eyes, and bones like bubble wrap – but your baby will be fine. So if all you can keep down for fifteen weeks is peanut butter and crackers, so be it. Baby will still be nourished.

A tip on nutrients for baby: Many women can't keep down those horse pills that smell like decaying yeast, otherwise known as the pregnancy multivitamin. If you can't keep it down, don't worry. Stop taking it and just pop a folic-acid pill once a day until the nausea passes.

As a theatre artist, work is sparse, and when it's there, time and money are so limited that you develop a Spartan work ethic. I have toughed through shows when I had strep throat, stomach flu, bronchitis, bleeding gashes, and really bad cramps. I did shows after funerals of loved ones. I've fainted on stage, recovered backstage, and got back on the boards.

Mind over matter is truly amazing. However, that implies a mind that is somehow on *your* side, instead of that grain-of-rice-sized freeloader's you're hosting. For the first time, my theatre work ethic failed me. I couldn't manage to do anything creative beyond making a spit-up bib out of my pyjama shirt.

At this point in the pregnancy, we came up with a nickname for our fetus. A very helpful Web site, www.babycentre.com, pointed out that this thing that was making me hurl my guts out was the size of a lima bean. From then on, our little one became known to all and sundry as "The Bean."

By week twelve, I was looking forward to a lessening of the symptoms. There was none. It was then that many women I spoke to admitted that morning sickness left them more around week fifteen or so. They don't tell you this when you're puking at week eight. No. Then they say, "You only have four more weeks of it." I think if they said, "You only have seven more weeks of it," more women would be convicted of murder.

This unfortunately is the best salve I have to offer: No matter how difficult your pregnancy turns out to be, it does end, and you will be you again — although a richer and more Amazonian survivor. And, with any luck, you'll be too busy to feel bad about anything that happened before your beautiful baby arrived.

BODY IMAGE

At first, I followed Ruth's advice and ate whenever I was nauseous. I hoped vainly that having food in my stomach would help me to stop heaving. That is how I ended up puking for eighteen weeks and still gaining weight. That, and the fact that the only things I wanted to eat were cheese and fries. Some books will tell you that you really don't need to gain anything for the first three months, or no more than five pounds. I always imagine that the people who offer these arbitrary weight goals are weedly thin men or women with pinched mouths and a disapproving "tch" constantly at the tip of their tongues. They iron their jeans. They have few friends and that's probably because they can eat whatever they want and they don't gain weight.

When I told my midwife, Sara, that I had put on twelve pounds already, she merely looked at me inscrutably and said, "Yes?" and waited for more. So I pressed on, "Well, that's a lot."

"Not really."

"I mean, shouldn't I be worried? Isn't that bad?"

She told me about the midwife from Denmark who had just visited their clinic. The Danish midwife was shocked that women were weighed every time they came for an appointment. Of course, the Danes show shock by murmuring, "Hmmmm." She said that in Denmark the women are never weighed. Her philosophy was: Who cares how much they gain, as long as they are healthy and their blood pressure, glucose, and protein levels are not too high.

I loved this attitude, and tried to abide by it. I felt full of feminist ire toward a society that values thinness so much that we tell pregnant women how much they "should" gain. Before I began to gain weight, I vowed that I would not be sucked in by the judgemental attitude that results in women being self-conscious at such a glorious and powerful time. I would not focus my energy on my appearance when I was creating life inside me! If my hormones wanted me to gain a hundred pounds, so be it!

Until Janis looked at me across the living room one day and called me her "chubby cutie." Apparently she thought I looked adorable with my double chin and puffy face.

I burst into tears. Janis instantly apologized and rushed to give me a hug, but got knocked back against a wall by a tremendous and liberating belch.

"I remember watching some TV show in my third month about pregnant models. Why, only God knows, but I'm watching this show and they all looked really cool in hip, clingy floral pants and midriff shirts with their big bellies sticking out saying, 'Hello, world, look at my stomach' and they were all sitting on a huge sofa giggling. I threw an orange at the screen and cracked it." – Robin, mother of twins

A provocateur director friend of mine, Alisa, dared me not to tell anyone I was pregnant for as long as I could, and just let the weight slowly creep up. She wanted to observe people around me saying, "Yeah, have you seen Flacks lately? She's really let herself go . . ."

There is one element of first trimester weight gain that makes it impossible to pretend that you are anything but pregnant. The boobs. It starts immediately. First, they are just sensitive and tingly. Pretty quickly, they start to grow. And grow.

One night I took off my shirt and tried to sneak into my pyjama jacket. Janis caught me and said, "Hold it! Let me look at you!" I froze. "Wow, did your breasts grow again in one day?" I looked in the mirror and it was someone else's body staring back at me. I felt weird, like this was some science-fiction story, and I was growing at a phenomenal rate. I almost didn't want to see my breasts. I felt out of control.

That is one of the toughest things for women to deal with. The lack of control. The fact that an animus, unconscious, personality-less, strong part of them was taking over. They had to just "let go" of everything, including their own bodies.

Robin advised not to bother letting go:

"Okay, soooo what's this ooga-booga good lesson about giving up control? DON'T EVER GIVE UP CONTROL. It's like people telling me to reduce my stress or tension. I like my stress and tension. It keeps me going. In fact I need it to survive, it keeps me in a constant state of disgust, an essential part of my personality and well-being."

As troubling as it is to be forced to contemplate losing control, it's good practice for being a parent: learning how to surf the chaos.

PREGNANCY SCARES

As mentioned in the previous chapter, many of us Jews have a tradition of not telling anyone the "news" until the second trimester because we are a paranoid and highly suspicious tribe and rightly so. We don't tell "just in case, God forbid, I hate to say it but ya never know, something should happen."

Sometimes something does. In my case, it happened during a night that Janis was up north visiting friends. After a fun-filled day of throwing up, I went to bed early. At 10:30 p.m. I started heaving. It went on until there was nothing left. I called Janis to come home. By midnight I was awakened by a bad stabbing pain in my gut. I lay on the bathroom floor. I reasoned that it was so laborious to lift my head that it was better to stay there. Also, I observed that I looked more pale and pathetic next to our cool blue tiling and maybe, like in a fairy tale, someone on a white horse would come and rescue me.

Janis arrived in her black rented truck around 1:00 a.m. and hoisted me up and back to bed. By 3:30 a.m. I was at it again. We started to worry that this wasn't just morning sickness. The stabbing pain was centred in my lower belly.

Not knowing what "normal" morning sickness entailed, we decided to call Telehealth Ontario, a new toll-free emergency help line. The optic-enhancing ads for it showed caring and well-rested young nurses offering instant aid. We dialled.

A nurse named Jennifer asked Janis for the correct spelling of her name, address, and postal code for their statistical records. Then she asked to talk to me. Janis said that I was throwing up at the moment, and maybe she could relay any information about my condition. Jennifer insisted she needed to talk to me personally. I wiped stomach acid from my chin and shakily took the phone. Jennifer asked me for the correct spelling of my name, my address, my postal code.

When I asked what could be wrong with me, Jennifer inquired as to how far along I was. "Eight weeks," I said. She paused and then replied that she couldn't really say what it was, and that it was best if I went to Emergency and let them take a look at me.

We got ourselves to the hospital and were sent to a triage nurse. Denise had sharp, ferretlike features, a tight grey ponytail, and a desperate desire to move things along. She told us in a real no-nonsense fashion that there would be a long wait, maybe six to eight hours. She asked how far along I was and when I said "eight weeks" she said it sounded to her like I was having an ectopic pregnancy. This occurs when the egg plants itself outside of the uterus, usually in the Fallopian tubes. She suggested that if we could find a gurney, I should lay down. We asked if we could be given priority because I was pregnant and she said she had people there with chest pains. Both Janis and my hearts were pounding as we stared the possibility of losing the baby in the face. That was the first moment that I realized how badly and how truly I wanted to have this child. Janis was stubbornly convinced that the nurse was wrong, and that I was going to be okay. I was not so sure.

Finally, we found a gurney and I fell asleep for a bit. I was later awakened by a nurse taking a blood test. Then back asleep to be awakened by them wheeling us into another section of Emerg. A brisk doctor came in, did a few listens with a stethoscope, felt my stomach, and said he'd be back when the lab had results from the blood tests. I held Janis's hand and we tried to squeeze our dire thoughts away. Janis distracted herself by becoming outraged with our doctor's flippant manner after we had waited so many hours to see him.

A few hours later, the brisk doctor returned and said the pregnancy was normal. We finally exhaled. It looked like it might be a bad case of the flu on top of severe morning sickness. He gave me a prescription for the anti-nausea drug Diclectin, assuring me it was designed for pregnant women and that his own wife took it. Then he leaned back, almost lounging against the counter, to answer any questions we had. He sighed that no one tells you how uncomfortable pregnancy is. His wife also had severe morning sickness. He called her a gladiator.

We got the pills, I took one, and we slept. This gladiator spent the next day on the sofa watching football and reading *People Magazine*. On the cover was a picture of Prince Edward and Sophie Rice Jones. She had just had an ectopic pregnancy. The focus of the article was about how no one visited her in the hospital. "Poor Sophie Rice Jones," I wept. (I also wept at an article about a dog who dials the phone for his blind owner.) I resolved to write Sophie a letter of support. But then my brain shrunk and I forgot.

"I had a pretty easy first trimester. No throwing up and I was still able to work. One day, I went for a long hike with the dogs and I felt so good, that I pushed it farther than I meant to. When I got home, I had intense cramps, and some blood spotting. I called my husband, Steve, at work, and was sobbing, 'It's my fault, I brought this on, I did this!' He called the midwife's office. They told me to lie down, not exert myself, and if the cramps or bleeding continued, to get to Emergency. Once I lay down, I fell asleep, and the spotting passed." – Netty

My second scare happened about a month later. After so many weeks of trudging about in an opaque vista of sickness, I awoke one early morning feeling quite normal. There was no whoosh whoosh of hormones, no fog, nausea, or dullness. Like when the air conditioning's been on for a while and you don't notice it. And then it suddenly shuts off, and everything is bright, loud, and clear.

I felt like me again for the first time in weeks. Was I happy about this reprieve? Of course not. I'm Jewish. I lay there for about an hour and a half silently panicking that this meant that the pregnancy was over. Finally I woke Janis up. "I don't feel anything."

"What? Well, that's good."

"No, I feel nothing. I feel like it's over." I started to wail. "It's my fault. I said I hated this."

It's true. The night before as I tried to answer Janis's question about what exactly I did all day, I actually said the words *I hate this*. I wanted her to feel and understand the nastiness of my state. I felt sick, uncomfortable, uneasy, unattractive, and uncaring. When I walked the dog, in my slow shuffle, old ladies left me in the dust. "You know what I do all day? I fart." I had wanted to be bad and tempt fate and act like a baby and not a mother and just complain. So now we were dealing with the repercussions of my evil impulses. What had my selfish thoughts manifested? No hormones were coursing through me. Those cranky old Hebraic superstitions were right!

Janis went on the Internet to www.babycentre.com to look up if you can suddenly stop having symptoms for no reason. I paced. Then suddenly I burped. Oh, I thought, that's a good sign. I burped again. Good. Very good.

Then, is this nausea I feel?

Then, a gag. YAH!

Janis peered into the hallway with hope in her eyes.

Suddenly I had two huge coughing gags and a small vomit. "YAHAHA!" I ran into the office and did a flailing, high-energy, celebratory jig, "I puked! I puked! Thank God!"

I squeezed my bloated, tender stomach, "I love you," I belched to my brave strong baby hanging on mightily despite me.

A tip: There's no mistaking it. This is a tough time. Don't feel the need to grin and bear it. I'd advise kvetching, seeking help, trying Diclectin for nausea. If you're one of those women who have no symptoms in this time, I bow to you because obviously you were a highly evolved soul in your previous life. Just try not to gloat around your grey, shuffling, farting, crying, gagging psycho pals. Or in the next life, you could come back as a grub.

4

The Second Trimester

What They Don't Tell You

Once I was showing, I suddenly noticed that pregnant women were everywhere: on the bus, in Swiss Chalet, at traffic court. Janis pointed out that they were always there, we just never gave a crap.

I recently had lunch with a woman who was coming out of her first trimester. She looked at me conspiratorially, "You know what they don't tell you?"

"What?" I whispered back equally furtively over a stack of creamers that my eighteen-month-old had erected and was in the process of destroying.

"Pregnancy is so much fun!" she hooted. My son bellowed, "Okay!" and a creamer exploded in his mouth.

While I wholeheartedly agree that being pregnant is one of the most joy-filled, awe-inspiring things a body can do, "fun" wasn't where I was at by week sixteen.

My lunchmate was aware of this and said, "You're sort of my benchmark. Nothing in my first trimester was as bad as yours, so I figured I was doing okay."

Glad I could help.

THE LIGHT

By week sixteen of my pregnancy, I had begun to chart days: barf (b), not barf (nb), partial barf (pb). I meticulously measured and recorded these details in a futile effort to weave order and control into the unpredictable tapestry that was my stomach.

Then, slowly, through a cluttered tunnel of charts and graphs, I realized that I was starting to see some light.

It began the day I took a ride on my bike to the corner store. While I had to lower the gears to "Grandma with a bad hip" levels, and I had to grunt and heave and sweat my way up my street (which was on a slight, but definite incline, something I was determined to complain to the city about) I made it to the store.

The only thing I can compare it to is when you have one of those long, ugly winter flus. You start to feel like you'll never have energy again, and you regret that you didn't really enjoy your life before. An endless wasteland of sick stretches before you. Until one day, you get a little pep back. Three days later, you forget what the flu was like.

Yet, I wanted to hold on to my experience of the first trimester. I was thrilled that I might get my personality back, but I didn't want to forget the magnitude of the change that had occurred in and to me.

I needn't have worried. The changes continued.

SHOWING BUT NOT SHOWING

The beginning of the second trimester is often marked by that odd phase of *showing, but not showing*. You're body is changing shape, but you don't have a pregnant belly yet. You might look a little puffy, plump, full. Let's be kind and say cherubic, zaftig, Rubenesque. Some women I know didn't put on an ounce until week twenty-two or so. But there was something different about them, if you looked closely enough. At their boobs.

If you've put on a few, as I had, you're in the interesting predicament of looking chubby but not pregnant. I got an audition

somewhere around week fifteen, when I could still "pass" as someone whose jeans must have shrunk in the dryer. I was conflicted
about going, because God knows casting directors think its a
bigger blow to your career to be fat than to be knocked up.

I went to a prenatal exercise class with Janis during this time.
We were standing in the bathroom looking in the mirror and I
whined that I couldn't wait to start showing and getting a belly
already. A woman next to us barely looked up from her hand-
washing to comment, "Oh, don't worry. You'll get big, all right!
Just *wait!*" She cackled maniacally and left. Janis and I rolled our
eyes and assured each other that that lady was a wacko.

From where I sit now, I'm sure that if I heard some barely pregnant woman complain that she wasn't big *enough*, I would
comment too. And I'm just slightly wacko.

Then, all of a sudden, you start to "pop out." The belly gets
round, and not just because of end-of-day bloat. The hips widen
and soon you won't be able to wear any of your pants – even the
super baggy ones – without feeling pulling in the crotch. Not a
good pulling.

Even if you're not really showing yet, my suggestion is to
get some maternity clothes. You may be able to borrow
some — I was lent some beautiful stuff. But do go
shopping and buy one or two things that fit you
specifically. I guarantee you will live in them. They're
designed for your body now, and you'll be chuffed with how
lovely you'll look in the right cut. How often are you
pregnant? Come on, drop some dough!

Once I was showing, I was thrilled. Suddenly I noticed that
pregnant women were everywhere: on the bus, in Swiss Chalet, at

traffic court. They had dogs, and other kids! It's like when you buy a Volkswagen and suddenly you notice all the Volkswagens on the road. I informed Janis of this revelation. "Look at all the pregnant women! It's a population explosion."

She pointed out that they were there before, we just never gave a crap. Now we blushed, smiled, and had intimate conversations with total strangers. "How far along are you? Are your nipples itchy?"

GETTING BIGGER

As you get bigger, people will start to touch you. Accept it. The belly must be rubbed like the magic lamp that it is. The general public acts like there is a genie inside there that will grant their wishes. *Your* wish might be that they stop *touching* you.

But I loved it. Pregnancy is tactile, sensual, hot, and primal. Touch seemed to be a more fitting way for people to acknowledge the feat we were undertaking than the classic Canadian nod 'n' smile 'n' dash.

I read a lot as I got bigger. I was so delighted to stop reading about puking that I joyfully dove into everything else. One or two of the books left a weird taste in my mouth. There was often a pseudo girlfriend-y, cheeky tone that implied:

"Honey, say goodbye to your body as you knew it."

"You may feel fat. You are."

"Men! They're so silly. You can't expect them to know what to do. You might as well tell *yourself* you're beautiful."

I felt smug and superior to these kinds of comments. I was like a teenager who had no sense of their own mortality. I believed that the things that happened to other mothers would not happen to me. My body would come back, my breasts would be fine, my relationship would only improve. Besides, I would not be someone who was preoccupied with her appearance during this miraculous time.

I've since discovered that even the most enlightened and analytical of women have trouble countering the negative messages in their heads about size, weight, appearance. Naomi Wolf notes this in her book *Misconceptions*: "As a heavy woman in society (I hoped temporarily, but who knew?) I felt as if I'd slipped several notches down in the social hierarchy of the world. My self-image had gotten skinned on the fast slide down . . ."

The billion-dollar industries that rely on women feeling bad about themselves, from fashion to diet to self-help, have managed to get into our heads and take a seat. The social structures that depend on women feeling "less than" have been working on us from the time we could talk. They certainly worked on me.

The following excerpts are from my pregnancy journal. A slice of what was going on inside my head and body. As you can see, I had good days when I welcomed the body changes: "Today I feel kind of ok like this is how I'm supposed to be, and kind of strutting it a bit. Maybe it's because I feel more like me in my body – except for the horrible gas. . . ."

And I had bad days when I felt alarmed and out of control: "I'm at seventeen weeks and I've put on twenty-five pounds! I feel so incredibly huge. I've never felt so out of control of my body. I'm trying not to panic. I wish I could work out more, but maybe if I can do aquafit twice a week and babyfit and yoga once it will help. Anyway, I'm obsessed and I feel terrible about it. When I meet new people I want to say, 'This is not the real me. Don't judge me by this size.' Does that mean I'm judging people all the time?"

In struggling with this dichotomy, a friend advised me to stop judging myself for the fact that I couldn't stop judging myself.

Weight is a heavy issue, pardon the pun. Many of us were chubby kids. Some of us have family histories of weight problems. Some of us work in industries where personal appearance is a factor in success. Some of us are simply freaked out by change. Or is that all just me? . . .

I had been trying to hold on to control with my fingernails. The first trimester somehow didn't succeed in teaching me that my body was not in my power any more. After all, much of how you'll look and what will happen to you is biologically predetermined. You may end up looking like a woman who swallowed a basketball, or you may look like my sister who resembled a woman who swallowed the great pumpkin, and then grew larger everywhere else to support it.

I am a short, short-torsoed, long-legged woman. I met a few other short-waisters at Prenatal Yoga one day who were very pregnant indeed. They said to get ready for the "barrel look." Instead of the bump in the lower belly, the short-waisted woman should prepare for the whole thing from chest down to become one big barrel. There is simply not a lot of room for the baby to go anywhere but out and around you.

I refused to believe that the barrel would happen to me; although I was beginning to accept that I would not resemble the aerodynamically sleek pregnant women that I saw on sitcoms. This was a glorious time of fecundity and I should have been proud of what my body could do. Instead I too often kneaded the flab on my legs, face, and arms and drew back.

In the public realm, I strutted my burgeoning self about with rapture. In my work life, I got activist. I wanted to put an image out there of what a real pregnant woman looked like, tumultuous tushie and all. I was more able to fight for another woman's right to be big, proud, and sexy than my own.

SEX AND THE BIG LADY

My pregnancy started off as a time when I wanted to kill my sexual partner for forgetting to close the lid to the garbage can.

The irony of feeling so disconnected from the person who knocked you up is rich. Never mind whether you feel attractive. If you have a kind partner, as I do, he or she will tell you that you look attractive. They may be lying. It doesn't matter. The point is, in the first few months, many women, even Scorpios like myself, do not remotely feel like doing it.

One night in those early weeks, I remember looking at my sleeping partner, feeling a great swell of love for her forbearance with me, the fact that she never complained or pushed me to go beyond what was comfortable or possible, and one very clear thought insinuated itself into my hormone-addled, sleep-deprived, upchuck-shook-up, nutrient vanquished brain: "YOU DID THIS TO ME!"

Thankfully, in the second trimester, Lady Libido spread her wings over our house and descended delicately back into our lives. She began by drifting into my dreams. They were vivid, and charged with the kind of painfully insistent sexuality I remember from my teen years. They were populated with exotic strangers and underwater exploits. I would wake flushed in a way I hadn't felt in months, maybe years, maybe never. Where the hell had I been all this time? Look who was right in front of me, closing the lid on the garbage can, mine for the taking!

The first time back from the long, cold gulag of trimester one did feel very much like a "first time." It was frantic, desperate, a great shock, a powerful secret — and over real fast. I cried. My first non-hormonal cry in weeks. I was suddenly painfully aware of how much I had needed to connect, to find some way of sharing what was going on in and for me.

As the second trimester progressed, the challenge became positioning. I asked myself, What do I do with these ginormous and ever-ballooning breasts? My nipples were big, dark bull's-eyes that seemed to attract more attention than before. Sometimes I even felt defensive for my old breasts, the small pink ones, a fading memory in the key of B cup. "Hey," I said, "those little champagne glasses were sexy too, weren't they?" Until the new heavy-duty breasts would respond with a shock that rocked me in a full-body wave, and I forgot to advocate for bouncy ounces any more.

One thing is for sure: the words *top* and *bottom* took on new meaning. You may be in the mood to be an aggressor in the sack, but not be able to manipulate yourself into anything but the most passive of supine postures. And vice versa: you may want to be taken in a bodice-ripping moment of submission, but on that day, heartburn might be so bad that you basically have to remain standing, with the most correct chiropractic alignment possible.

Oddly, the bigger I got, the more I wanted to do it. And I'm not the only one.

A friend told me about the women with whom she shared a long hospital stay in the last few months of her delicate and difficult pregnancy. One dreary day they all got to talking about sex. Some were not into it at all. Some felt dirty, looking at their huge wiggling bellies and feeling ashamed about how this happened to them. Some were libidinous Wonder Women craving the next moment when their stud would arrive and they could close the curtain for a conjugal visit. And one woman who was carrying twins discovered a neat little trick. If she sat up at just the right angle, the weight of her belly rolling forward would make her climax. Just like that. It was an incredible discovery and once she found it, she did it. A lot. Now that's nature's way of creating balance, justice, and harmony.

EXERCISE

One of the other great joys of the second trimester was being able to get my creaky bones active again.

I joined a class called Baby and Me Fitness. The class was supposed to be for pregnant women, but it turned out to be mostly new moms. The instructor set a bunch of mats up in the middle of the floor. The moms put the babies down on their backs and we all exercised around them.

Looking down at these needy, blobby, crying creatures, and their attentive, fragmented, harried moms I suddenly grasped that these women couldn't even scrounge forty-five minutes a week to work out on their own. A naked thought streaked across my mind, And just what are these women getting *back* from their babies?

I was used to pushing myself, really muscling through and into the workout. So when the first trimester ended, I was back to doing men's pushups and squats. I spent the gentle, supportive Baby and Me Fitness classes grunting away, testing myself, showing off, desperately trying to be as fit as I believed I should be. Struggling against the vision of those women who were now merely vassals chained to the servitude of their needy babies. Well, my macho workouts didn't last long. My balance was off, my centre of gravity had dropped, and my joints were turning me into Gumby (and Pokey). It became clear that I may have felt better, but I was not who I used to be. I had to find a gentler and less high-impact form of exercise. I joined prenatal yoga. It was one of the best things I've ever done.

Pigeon Pose – Yoga Mama

Before I was pregnant, you could not drag me to a yoga class. Internal calm and other people's moist, naked feet make me nervous. However, three months of moving from the bed to the couch to the toilet had taken its toll on my body. I knew I needed to get grounded, in touch, and gently stretched or I risked injuring myself as I got back to semi-normal activity – like sitting up.

The yoga studio that I chose to go to was picked by fluke. An instructor from the Yoga Space had come to the play that I was doing at the time that I got pregnant. She offered a free class to each member of the cast. I chose the Yoga Space, which is all the way across town from me, because it was free.

As it turns out, it is run by doulas. Wonderful, irreverent downtown doulas. Doulas are non-medically certified prenatal, labour, and postnatal assistants. Most often, they ascribe to the natural childbirth school. They teach breathing, different labouring positions.

They encourage expression of fears and hopes. Some will also help around the house after the birth and with breastfeeding. They are there to fill a void in our modern, medically mandated system. Janis and I already had that in a midwife, so we didn't choose to use a doula. Still, I did hang around after class twice a week to ask them dozens of odd, embarrassing questions like, "Could that be the baby's foot digging into my Vajuj?"

The class was surprisingly fun. It made us expectant moms feel special, and that pregnancy was a sacred thing. It was also a space where we could talk about our gas. I felt instant sisterhood with a group of women that I had just met.

The first class I attended happened to be full of women who were pretty far along. I felt like a bit of an imposter – little old chubby but not showing me. At first the other women looked right through me, thinking I was there for something else. When they realized I was in the correct class and was pregnant, intimacy erupted, "Do your breasts feel tingly? Do you ever get a weird twinging in the muscles between your labia, or is it just me?"

As I started to discuss my pussy lips with a complete stranger, a tall, blonde, gigantic woman waddled excitedly up to me and exclaimed, "Diane, are you pregnant?"

I had no idea who she was.

"Fourteen weeks," I said, as automatically as a soldier's name, rank, and serial number. I racked my brain.

Noting my poorly disguised look of confusion, she explained, "I know. I'm huge. The last time you saw me we had just started trying to conceive."

The penny finally dropped. Fiona was an actress who had been in a short play that I wrote for a fundraiser. At that very moment, I realized that I had never seen a nine-and-a-half-month pregnant woman in the flesh before. I had no idea how *big* a pregnant woman could get. Fiona was abundant. Extravagant. Luscious. Terrifying. I murmured to myself, "Well, I won't get *that* big."

Aquafit

During my pregnancy I became quite a joiner. Besides yoga and Baby and Me, I joined an aquafit class.

I was snobby at first. I assumed I'd be in a pool with a bunch of old *bubameisahs* and people with fused spines – dog paddling in slow motion to the echo-y strains of Billy Joel. The classes turned out to be pretty tough. By the end, I could barely waddle my way through. Yet, just being in water was a delight, as my mother would say, "What a *mechiya!*" Without gravity schlepping on me I felt agile, strong, liberated.

There was one way that the class was not liberating. In order to do the exercises, we wore belts around our waists to keep us afloat. As I got bigger, the belt had to move higher and higher, ending up in the half-inch space between my boobs and my ribs. You *could* call that a waist, but it wasn't meant for a belt. The pressure of the belt and the effect of the water's buoyancy on my stomach caused tremendous heartburn. During one class I had to quickly make my way over to the side of the pool to burp and swallow while everyone else was cross-country skiing under the water to Cindy Lauper's "She Bop." The instructor saw me in distress and came over, flushed with the prospect of using her Emergency training. I regretted to inform her that I just needed a moment to belch "O Canada!" and I'd be fine. She shrugged, disappointed, and moved on to underwater bike-pedalling.

I have no idea if all the yoga, walking, and aqua-womaning helped me during labour. Or if keeping my body somewhat toned facilitated recovery and weight loss after childbirth. It did contribute to finding my equilibrium. It was also a real kick to get naked and shower my big body in a room full of other women. I'd linger in the hot water, letting anyone who wanted eyeball the Bean Pod. I never felt so uninhibited in my life. I think I actually preened. I felt like a luxurious, urban Venus, comfortable under the gaze of her tiny admirers.

The Second Trimester • 73

IT'S *MY* BABY IN *ME* – FIRST MOVEMENTS

This is the fun part. The profoundly wondrous revelation. All the nausea and weight gain is actually in aid of something. With every flurry of activity, each burst of feeling, I fell madly in love with my brave little being, just hanging out inside me, living its own life.

Within an incredibly short time period you will go from you alone being able to feel the baby moving inside you – to anyone being able to feel it from the outside – to being able to *see* the baby's clearly articulated body parts bouncing around its snug, living house.

The Bean's first movement occurred around eighteen weeks. I was sitting in a writers room with a bunch of very quick-witted men (I was the only female writer in the room). We were working on a television sketch series. A comedy writers room can be a pretty competitive arena, with snappy lines flying fast and furious. I generally challenge myself to get in there with as much testosterone as I can muster. But in this room, I found myself merely acting as "The Feeder": the one whose job is basically to laugh at other people's jokes and repeat them, "Titsy Von Assonher, that's a funny name . . ."

At one vital meeting as we were getting closer to production, we were discussing the reaction of a network executive to our first read-through. The guys were getting heated, "Yeah, well, they don't like it because they don't *get* it."

"Exactly – it's a prison romance."

"*That's* funny."

"Yeah!"

There was one other woman in the room – a producer, Lynne, who had two kids. I interrupted the coffee-fuelled fussing.

"Yeah, yeah, I know what you mean about the network and the prison thing, but um, Lynne, did the first baby movement feel like a little flip?"

Her eyes opened wide, "Yes!" she exclaimed.

The room full of crusty comics burst into applause. I said, "I wasn't sure if it was the baby or last night's hummus." I got a laugh. That was the best laugh my sluggish wit incited on that job.

After the flips, you'll feel kicks. What does a kick feel like? It feels like a kick. As the baby gets bigger, it can really knock your socks off. But in the beginning, it's little nudges and tickles. Love taps. And then it's Love KOs.

"The first kick seemed to come early. We saw the seatbelt go boop! And we both laughed with the joy of it all. Life was good." – Lily, mother of three, safta (grandmother) of Eli

"We felt our daughter's first kick during a night out at the symphony. The concert was Tchaikovsky's *Romeo and Juliet*. We're watching closely to see if she becomes a musician or a hopeless romantic." – Nancy and Charles, parents of one

Janis felt The Bean kick for the very first time around week twenty-two or so. I had been feeling it for a few days from the inside. We were lying in bed, and I could suddenly feel it from the outside. I grabbed her hand and pushed it forcefully onto the spot I'd just felt kicking. We waited. The kick moved somewhere else. Damn. I wouldn't give up. I chased that kicker down with Janis's palm. Finally, she felt it. "Aha!" I smiled into her face – thrilled with this amazing gift that I could now share with her. I expected her to burst out laughing or crying. Instead, she mumbled, "Whoa. Weird," her brows knitting together in shock.

She confessed that it was a bit disconcerting to her. There was a living being that I was growing inside my body. Kind of like the movie *Alien*. I looked at her as if *she* was the alien. To me, this had already become the most natural thing in the world. Besides, what did she think was in there all this time? Jello?

After feeling the kick, Janis worried that it might be uncomfortable for me. She said that people had told her that it gets so bad you can't sleep, what with the baby's little elbow digging into your rib cage. The kicks never got that way for me. I loved the movement even when I felt like I was being sucker-punched from the inside.

Yes, it does sucker-punch you. Luckily, in the early days of my second trimester, I often got some warning. I would feel like something was going to happen. A stirring inside, maybe it was the amniotic fluid sloshing around, and then boom-boom soccer baby!

Before you can feel your baby spiralling, kicking, and floating around, you will probably hear it.

LISTEN UP! I'M IN HERE!

At my first appointment with my midwife after trimester one, she asked me if I'd like to hear the baby's heartbeat.

"Would I?!"

She brought out the machine that became my absolute favourite medical implement of all time, surpassing the stethoscope and those cool instant thermometers that go in your ear: the Doppler machine. This little device picks up the sound of the baby's heartbeat and amplifies it to fill the whole room: the Doppler rocks!

Sara, the midwife, squeezed some gel on my stomach, placed the wand of the Doppler on my belly, and started looking for the baby. I could hear my own heartbeat in a sea of shooshing whale sounds. My heartbeat was a slow "woop . . . woop . . . woop."

The longer Sara searched for the baby's heartbeat without finding it, the faster my "woops" became. I silently panicked. Sara explained that my uterus was still below my pubic bone, making it hard to find the baby.

Although I was relieved to know this, the news that my uterus was still below my pubic bone was a bit of a blow to me because my stomach was already sticking out quite a bit. I had to accept that the bulge wasn't baby, it was French fries.

Then I heard it. First there was my "woop . . . woop . . . woop . . ." and then a fast, bouncy "dut dut dut dut dut dut!" There it was! Right there! Beating away! Our baby strong and loud!

I was so proud. This new being was working away at living. Who knew at what moment its soul would arrive – or had arrived? And it was asserting itself so brilliantly in the world already. You go, rocking Bean. You *go*!

By my next appointment the following month, my uterus had popped up front and centre above my pubic bone. Before the midwife could get the Doppler six inches from my belly, we heard The Bean's grooving "dut dut dut dut dut." I burst into tears and laughter. "Thank you, little one," I murmured. "I know. I know you're here."

NICE TO SEE YOU

The next big milestone in the "it's really real!" journey was seeing the baby on an ultrasound.

We were booked by our midwives into an ultrasound that would aid in our decision-making about whether to do amniocentesis. Since I was thirty-five, there was an increased risk statistically that I could have a child with Down syndrome or another form of chromosomal abnormality.

As part of genetic testing, we decided to do a new ultrasound at thirteen weeks called nuchal translucency. During this ultrasound, the thickness of the folds in the back of the neck of the fetus is measured. The thicker the folds, the higher the possibility of Down or other chromosomal abnormality.

Nuchal translucency, also known as the thirteen-week ultrasound, was a relatively new test that had better accuracy than the more common blood tests called triple screen. Many of my friends had had the triple-screen blood test done and got a positive result for genetic birth defects.

> "After the positive blood test, we booked amniocenteses to make sure. My husband and I were told there was a $1/200$ statistical rate of miscarriage as a result of amnio. Our doctor said that this was just an average and that many of those miscarriages occurred in high-risk pregnancies. We had to wait two to four weeks for the results. During which time we rarely slept, and basically were *fahrmished* – in knots." – Rachel, mother of two

By the time the results came in, they were feeling baby movement. So any decision that they might have to make, should the amnio also come back positive for a serious problem, would be made under the backdrop of having felt their baby kicking.

In Rachel's case, the amnios were negative. So the false-positive triple-screen blood tests succeeded in prompting her to do the invasive amnio for no reason. We decided not to take the triple-screen blood tests at all. We relied on the more accurate thirteen-week ultrasound.

Before we had it done, we discussed how we felt should the ultrasound indicate that my risk was high for a child with chromosomal abnormality. Janis was convinced that we could handle anything that came our way. I was not so sure. I questioned my ability to be a competent mother to a *healthy* child.

We had the ultrasound at a hospital in downtown Toronto. From the friendly and always informative environment of the midwifery clinic, we were suddenly crowded into a waiting room with dirty bathwater–coloured walls and carpets, packed with dozens of other couples at different stages of pregnancy. The room reminded me of being in a large bus, at rush hour, in the summer. There were rows of seats, all facing the same way, and they were packed. Very buslike BO permeating the room (every-one there had an understandably nervous pong).

To deal with my boredom, and anticipation, I immediately and compulsively started comparing my girth to everyone else's.

"Do I look bigger to you than that chick over there with the shoulder pads and the stirrup tights?" I whispered to Janis as she tried to read a *Parenting* magazine from 1998.

"No, sweetie, you're – oh actually, yes you are. She must be here for another test."

She was. She was there for the *eighteen*-week ultrasound! She was a month farther along than I was.

Luckily, before I could further indulge my self-consciousness, another more urgent feeling made its presence keenly felt.

In preparation for this ultrasound, you are asked to drink a litre of water and not pee. This helps bloat your bladder and push the uterus to a better position for viewing. In effect, they make your bladder gigantic and bursting and then they sit there pressing on it with the ultrasound wand.

"The best was when one of the nurses told me I had too much fluid and I should just go pee some of it out. Well you can imagine that once I started peeing there was no way to stop." – Michelle, mother of three

Despite the three-hour wait and the bursting bladder, Janis and I were bubbling with excitement. We would finally get to see our Bean!

We were led into a tiny, dark room with a gurney and a table with the ultrasound monitor and equipment. Janis hovered by my side. Blue gel was plopped on my stomach, and our technician started pressing away. On a monitor, psychedelic images danced around like a living lava lamp. The technician uh-huh-ed her way through this human soup, making sense of an acid trip. "Look, there's its hands," she mumbled. For a brief flash, we saw something that looked like rigatoni.

"Wow, are you feeling a lot of movement?" the technician asked.

"Not really," I responded, gritting my teeth as I tried not to tinkle.

"This little one is flipping like crazy. Oh, now it's hiding from me. Can you cough please and we're see if it'll jump back around?"

All we could see was what looked like a flipping curled-up baby bird. That was in me?

"You've got a busy jumping bean in there," the technician said as she wiggled the wand about my belly.

"That's our Bean!" I said, giving Janis's hand a happy squeeze.

"Yup. You're in for it with this one," our technician chuckled.

We chuckled too, but I shot Janis a "what does that mean?" look.

Finally, after the measurements were done, she gave us the tour. She froze the monitor on an image.

"That string of pearls is its spine. Here are its hands and feet." She took some snapshots of The Bean in different positions to give to us for later.

Next we waited in a little room for the results. We were somberly reminded why we were there as we scanned the literature that detailed some of the diseases they could test for.

A doctor came in with a questionnaire. She asked me whether my husband's family had any history of genetic diseases. I told her that the baby's father was not my husband, and there were no genetic diseases.

"Oh, I'm sorry, your partner," the doctor corrected herself.

Janis and I hadn't felt like coming out to the whole department if it wasn't necessary. Until the doctor pointed to Janis and added, "Your sister can stay with you while you wait for the results."

"She's my partner."

The doctor flushed. "Oh. I see. Sorry. Congratulations to you both." She backed out of the room.

Janis's face was red. We held hands. She told me I didn't have to do that if I didn't want to.

"No *way* are you going to be invisible," I fumed. "This is your child. You're Bean's mommy. Let them *try* to ignore you!"

Then another doctor, older, very conservative-looking, came in to give us our results. He shook my hand. I immediately and defensively introduced Janis, my *partner*, ready to ask him to step outside. He shook her hand and sat. Clearly, he could care less. I loved him instantly. He told us that for my age, the odds of chromosomal abnormalities are about $1/250$. The numbers they got for me from the ultrasound were $1/1,520$. The risk factor of a fifteen- or twenty-year-old. I wanted to kiss the guy. We were spared the agony of the amnio and its associated decision-making.

I bragged about my low-risk factor for weeks. I sounded a lot like David and his "pretty big cupful of spunk today, huh?"

EIGHTEEN-WEEK ULTRASOUND
Five weeks later, we had another ultrasound. The eighteen-week comprehensive ultrasound. The last ultrasound test we had for the duration of the pregnancy. At eighteen weeks, the baby is big enough that all its limbs and organs can be seen, but not too big that some of its body could be hidden from the screen.

This test would really let them have a look at our child and indicate any abnormalities with everything from fingers to kidneys. We were excited to observe our little Bean, but the nerves were there too. How much do we want to know if there is a problem? What would we do about it?

Again I was told to drink and not pee. Once more the ultrasound technician's wand flamencoed on and around my bladder. But this time, the baby was much more real-looking.

The technician asked, "Do you want to know the gender?"

"No," I replied.

"Yes," said Janis simultaneously.

I whipped my head around, "What?!"

"Well," Janis shrugged, "it's right there. We could know. Wouldn't that be wild?"

"I don't *think* I want to, but . . . ," I vacillated.

"Mama wins," said the technician and moved on. "See this string of pearls . . ."

At one point, the technician and baby held still. The Bean was on its side, tiny hands playing with tiny feet. Then, slowly, The Bean's head turned toward the monitor. The Bean looked right at us. Big lightbulb-shaped head and huge oval eyes. Calm stare. We gasped. The technician assured us that all babies look like E.T. at this stage.

But that wasn't what got to me. It was a feeling. Like The Bean was saying, "Yes, it's me. And you are? . . ."

GENDER

Every time I heard the heartbeat, I believed that The Bean was a girl. This was probably because someone told me that a fast heartbeat means a girl. When I mentioned this to the midwife, she said that all babies at this early stage have fast heartbeats.

Janis was convinced from the beginning that it was a boy.

I didn't want to know for a number of reasons. One was the way that people, even unconsciously, begin to gender-type a baby from the time it's a fetus. We'd already heard, "You're not painting the room mauve are you? What if it's a boy?!"

If we knew the gender for sure, we'd really hear it. Every choice of decor, attitude, or outfit would have to be gender-appropriate, or we'd endure all sorts of regressive, panicked pronouncements. I always wanted to put some perspective to these preoccupied people, "What's the worst that could happen? His yellow hat could make him gay? Hello! Big old pregnant dykey-dyke here, right in front of ya! And I'm doing okay!"

"I can't forget the yucky sexist stuff how if you look good pregnant you are having a boy and if you don't it's because a girl steals your looks." – Michelle, prenatal yoga pal and mother of two

I was certainly sick of people dissecting my body to indicate the gender of the baby. Carrying low, carrying high, spreading out in front, behind, underneath.

I recently heard this conversation between a pregnant woman and a total stranger:

"Are you expecting a boy or a girl?" Asked the nosy stranger, let's call her N.S.

"I don't know," said the pregnant woman, let's call her P.W.

"Let me see your hands," commanded N.S.

P.W. lifted her hands, as instructed.

"It's a boy," concluded N.S. instantly. "If you hold your hands palm up, you're carrying a boy, palm down it's a girl."

"Who told you that?" asked the incredulous P.W.

"My dental hygienist," replied N.S.

"I'm not exaggerating when I say that over a hundred people at work felt the urge to stagily stop me in mid-stride, inspect my belly, and make an authoritative statement about the gender of my child. They overwhelmingly decided I was having a boy (only two guessers said girl). Of course Madeleine was born with all her girl parts. Later when I went to visit the workplace to show off the baby, some showed a flicker of disappointment. I'm still not sure if they were expressing a preference for a male child or were disappointed that they had guessed wrong." – Nancy, midwife-group buddy and mother of one

I have to admit that the deeper reason I didn't want to know the gender of our Bean was because of my own potential for changing *my* behaviour or disposition toward our tiny bundle of possibility. Part of me felt that since we were two women, it might be easier if we had a girl. I was worried that if I found out it was a boy early on, a tiny chemical strand of "shucks" might be absorbed and understood by my child. I did not want The Bean to feel anything but joy and excitement from either of us. So I preferred not to know, hoping that whatever we had, we would be smitten by the time s/he arrived. Now, I couldn't imagine *not* having my beautiful little boy!

NEW SYMPTOMS

"I remember being very emotional, sweating all the time, peeing all the time, and figuring I could eat everything in sight because 'I would have to lose the weight afterwards anyway.'" – Michelle, mother of three

Heartburn

Once the vomiting of the first trimester ended, I immediately started having heartburn. For some reason I believed that you shouldn't take Tums during pregnancy. I think I was mistakenly told this by one of the thousands of people that lobbed "truisms" at me.

Receiving well-meaning but totally screwed-up advice is one of the disadvantages of starting to show. In my mother's generation, there were some doozies.

"An older woman whom I did not know came over to congratulate me. She then told me not to raise my hands above my head, as then the chord would choke the baby." – Lily

I was being a real purist in my pregnancy – no booze, no caffeine, no smoking, no Brie cheese or shellfish *ever*. I treated these "bad things" like biblical adversaries, to be shunned completely.

So due to my own orthodoxy in observance, I suffered needlessly through the heartburn. It can get pretty burpy and intense. Your stomach is being squished, which forces acid up your throat. Progesterone causes the sphincter muscle between the stomach and esophagus to remain partially open, which allows acid reflux. (Did you know you *had* a sphincter in your throat? It gives new meaning to the phrase *sounding like an asshole*.)

The mucous linings of your esophagus (and elsewhere) are also getting mushier due to the hormones flowing through you. This is one of the reasons you may start to pee when you laugh. Then pee when you gasp at the fact that you've peed. Then pee when you try to scoot to the bathroom. Words of advice: Don't scoot. Just have some Tums.

"Juicy Hips"

The hormones may also make you feel like your hips are on ball bearings. Your joints will be all loose and juicy. (Yes, *juicy* is the technical term.) This is caused by the secretion of the hormone relaxin. Relaxin's job is to loosen the tendons and ligaments, especially in the hips, so that they can be stretched open more easily in labour. It results in a slack-limbed feeling. I often felt like my hip bones were sliding into new positions as I walked. Your feet may become (and remain) wider as the tendons stretch. You might also develop a little back pain or sciatica as joints get shifted and stretched, and press on your nerves. Metaphorically and literally.

Midnight Leg Cramp

A bizarre symptom to arrive was the midnight leg cramp. If I so much as pointed my toe one millimetre in my sleep, my calf would seize up and I'd have to bolt (in slow-motion pregnancy pace) out of bed. I'd hop about like a gigantisaurus, yelping, stretching my heel, and massaging my calf. I was advised to eat a banana before bed to get more potassium into my system. That usually resulted in some banana burping to accompany my charley-horse jitterbug. The causes of leg cramps are not really known. The midwives guess that it's due to poor circulation and nerve compression because of the enlarged uterus. So, in other words, ain't much you can do.

"Crazy Eyes"

I also experienced an interesting change that I noticed in other women. It was in the eyes. Every single picture that was taken of me from the first week through to week forty-one had a similar feature. We called it "crazy eyes." I had a freaky fire-behind-the-eyes look to me. Not unlike a religious fanatic or Charles Manson. Try as I might to relax them, my eyes popped out. The right bigger than the left. Whatever expression I was trying to convey was outshone by these beacons of dementia. In person, people commented that my eyes were clear and bright. This is something that I saw immediately with my sister and many of my friends. It's a beautiful perk that seems to glow with some of the force of the little life inside you. But on film I looked like a mad scientist.

Skin Changes

Your skin will become more sensitive. My sister got rashes that came and went inexplicably. Some women develop a patch on their face of darker pigment. It's referred to as a "mask of pregnancy." I decided that if I developed this symptom I would wear a "Nixon mask of pregnancy" just for fun.

Some women start growing more hair on their skin. The hair on their head becomes thicker, wilder, more primal. Think of the huge, teased heads of hair on those 1980s glam rock bands like Twisted Sister or on the always reliable Cher.

Your nipples will get darker. If they're brown, they'll get more brown, and if they're pink, they'll turn chocolate. This was explained to me as nature's way of painting a bull's eye on the baby's food source. Newborns can't see very well. So the darker your nipple is in contrast to your skin, the easier it will be for them to find it and chow down. I would like to have this distinguishing feature incorporated in my pantry so that I can find the chips behind the old oatmeal and soya crap.

Many women get a *linea negra*, a dark line down the centre of the stomach from belly button to sternum. I have no idea what this is about. I used to joke that the line marks where the zipper will be. I patiently explained to people, "Nature will provide a zipper down my belly along this line. Just like She's made me grow matted troll hair and have crazy eyes. I'll simply unzip and the baby will come out, right? No pain, no fuss. How civilized."

Emotional Equilibrium – HAH!

Good news! The moods from trimester one continue! You may be somewhat back to your normal life, and feel more like yourself, but I had many days when the tears would just not stop. I cried at Bell commercials, reruns of *Seinfeld*, and any birthday card with an animal on it. I was fully aware that I had lost all perspective. But awareness and acceptance are two different things.

In my first trimester, my personality had changed in order to cope with the vomiting, but by the second trimester, I realized the changes were entrenching themselves. I was weepy, I'd developed a persecution complex, I was self-involved, I was ferociously short-fused (fer fuck's sake!) Moreover, I became very, very protective.

During a prenatal yoga class, a penny dropped that made profound sense. I was lying on my little blue mat at the end of a difficult class. We all had our eyes closed. We were in Shavasana, a sometimes endless two or three minutes of quiet relaxation. Suddenly I realized that the instructor was moving around in the room. I peeked. She was going up to each person in the class and massaging their faces with lavender oil. She came to me. I admit, it made me uptight. Dear God, she was about to touch my face with her fingers, and who knows where they'd been! I felt guilty for being tense. I didn't want her to think her class had failed to relax me. I tried to keep perfectly still, and pretend that I was a calm and confident person who openly accepted her healing touch. My eyelids were fluttering and twitching and every part of me was clenched.

After she was gone, I took a deep breath, relaxed, and put my hands on my belly. I felt a little pip of something pressing into my palm, as if to say, "Chill, Mama." The instructor finally spoke, "Yoga is about unity, of mind and body. You are all uniting with your babies in your bodies." In a flash, I felt it: this is not just *a* baby that will be coming into our lives. It's *my* baby. It's in *me*. I vowed, as the tears steamed into my ears, that I would do everything in my power to protect it.

From that moment, something shifted in me. I knew that The Bean at this stage was affected by bright lights, loud noises, bitter and sweet tastes. S/he could hear my heartbeat. So I refused to consider any work that might be stressful. I abruptly ended upsetting conversations. I once hung up on an obviously emotionally disturbed colleague with the words, "I'm having a baby! Don't call me again!" Suddenly nothing mattered more than maintaining some equilibrium for the baby. I chose The Bean.

Janis has a different perspective on this change. She describes it as me suddenly, and for The Bean's sake, developing a "good" intolerance, a "healthy" impatience. If anyone had a problem with that – my attitude was no longer "Oh no, what did I do?" It was now "Too bad. The Bean's first."

When my son was about two years old, I happened to be talking about this emotional protectiveness to three grandmothers. As I spoke, I couldn't help but experience residual guilt – maybe I *had* been unfair to my friends, too emotional, too precious. One of the women, Siobhan, a grandmother of three, flashed her pale blue eyes at me and said, "Every animal in nature has the instinct to protect its young. It's natural and right. No one should be foolish enough to challenge a pregnant woman in any way, emotionally or otherwise, that would compromise her baby." The other women nodded their heads sagely, as if it was the most obvious thing in the world.

If you value your relationship with a pregnant woman, do not put her in a position where she feels the need to protect her Bean or Sprout or Grain of Rice. She's not the same emotionally as she was. You might get hurt.

Paradoxically, acting "the same" despite the obvious emotional and physical changes that a pregnant woman is enduring seems to be a highly valued trait to some people, especially employers. How often have you heard comments like these:

"She worked until the day before she went into labour."

"She was sending faxes from the delivery room!"

"What a trooper!"

As I listened to these kinds of pseudo complements, I realized that pregnant women were not valued for what they actually *were doing*: simply being pregnant. They needed more room than they were getting emotionally, socially, in employment. They needed not to be judged by a male-defined standard of toughness. They deserved to be treated like the queens they are. I wanted to scream, "They're kinda busy with a vital twenty-four-hour-a-day job. Cut them some slack!"

Carpal Tunnel

A friend of mine developed carpal tunnel syndrome in her second trimester. Carpal tunnel involves pain and numbness in the major nerve of the hand and wrist. I always thought of it as an old person's disease. Like so many other pregnancy-related symptoms – from back pain to incontinence.

One day in my yoga class, our instructor, Kathryn, was commenting about how tough it is to meditate when you're pregnant because you have so much going on in your brain and body. Then she asked if anyone was having any particular pains. A red-haired woman, Sarah, with a torpedo-shaped belly, mentioned that she had terrible carpal tunnel in her wrists and she was in tons of pain. "But I'm due in four days so I hope it will be over soon."

A reed-thin blonde woman who looked about four months along – but was actually seven – piped up, "Don't be so sure. I had to have surgery!" Her carpal tunnel started after her first baby was born and she still had pain and weakness, now pregnant with number two.

So Sarah said, "Well, my doctor told me that with cases this severe, it should pass after birth."

"Just be careful," warned Reedy, "when you're picking up your baby or anything. Mine started because of using the breast pump! They just don't tell women about this. I had to have surgery and it's still painful, so that's all I'm saying is watch out."

This went back and forth a bit longer. The pain was described a little more. The whole room was listening in a kind of quiet terror, everyone's mind reeling with dread.

When the conversation ended, I whispered, "And now . . . meditate."

That broke the ice and we laughed. Then we all stampeded to the bathroom to pee.

Appetite

Many women describe a ravenous, sickening hunger – a desperate need to eat *immediately*. Like other pregnancy symptoms, it may remind you of the worst of your PMS. The drive to eat that Kit Kat in one bite is wildly intense, and not to be trifled with. If I didn't eat every few hours, something with protein (or chocolate), I would feel like passing out and barfing.

I succumbed to these urges. Besides not being able to fight them, I think there was a part of me that just wanted to go for it. Everyone told me that this was the one time in life when I could eat that extra piece of chocolate cake. It was a relief and a bit of a naughty thrill to just have dessert, fer fuck's sake.

As Naomi Wolf says in *Misconceptions*, "Some women were happy to be 'permitted' to eat normally for the first time in their adult lives."

Of course, it can get carried away, as this e-mail that I wrote in my fifth month illustrates:

"Stop me, please! I just bought a brownie mix. (It might have been low-fat brownie mix, but it's not going to help if I eat the whole pan, which I WILL.) Last night I dreamt I was at an all-you-can-eat burrito buffet. When I got there, there were thirty different kinds of baba ghanouj. There was also an all-you-can-eat tart buffet. I know, I know, I *am* an all-you-can-eat tart buffet . . .
p.s. I had a dream that the baby was a girl. What do you think of the name 'Clara'?"

The dreams during pregnancy were like Imax movies of the unconscious. I was surrounded by sensation. One night I dreamt that the skin of my stomach was made of thin, flimsy plastic, like a balloon. Janis was trying to hug me, but in so doing was crushing the baby. I yelled at her, "Get away from me and the baby!"

In our daily lives I was becoming more dependent on Janis, physically and emotionally. I couldn't imagine feeling so protective of the baby that I would want Janis to get away. I only needed to wait until the baby was born to understand the complex truth in this dream. And I didn't have much longer to wait.

● ● ●

A trimester-two tip: Strut, strut, and strut. And when you're done, prance. This time is a little parcel of glory, so revel, sister.

● ● ●

5

The Third Trimester

Gimme Room!

Every so often you must stop and loudly
say "Oy," even if you're not Jewish.

I loved my third trimester even more than the second. I felt like I was finally getting accustomed to the rapid changes that happen during pregnancy. I revelled in getting really big. I took tons of nudie pictures of my belly and boobs and e-mailed them inadvisably to too many people.

We were into late spring and summer and I was walking and exercising and enjoying people's delight and other parents' shared joy. I felt a giddy communion with other pregnant women and mothers. I didn't even mind perfect strangers touching my belly. Half the time I was willing to let them cop a feel of the "girls" too.

There are a few things, though, that we need to discuss. Things that can make the third trimester smooth or rough. And when you're carrying dozens of pounds of new life around, you want it as smooth as possible.

NAMES

We were superstitious about coming up with names until we were more or less out of the woods for the possibility of a miscarriage. So we waited to discuss it seriously until the third trimester.

We wanted a name with meaning. One that implied noble characteristics that our child could ascribe to him- or herself. A name also honours family members. Luckily, in the Jewish tradition, you can only name a child after someone who is already dead. Someone who can't kvetch to be a first name instead of a middle.

A name is a tender thing. It is wrapped up with purpose, resonance, cultural echoes, familial remembrance, pretty sounds. It can be easily crushed, so beware of telling too many people the name too soon.

Janis and I were at a brunch near the end of my third trimester and we were asked what names we'd picked out. We looked at the kind, expectant, eager faces of our friends smiling at us from across the patio table. We decided to share. We mentioned the girl names first. We spoke in hushed and reverent tones, as if exposing a baby bird to the light.

"Ruby. Clara. Sara."

We looked around at our friends' faces. There was silence.

"Those are old-fashioned names."

"I know *so* many Saras."

"What are your boy names?"

For a boy, we had even fewer options. Okay. We had one. Raphael in Hebrew means healed by God. It sounds musical and can be said in many different languages.

"You can call him 'Raffi,'" mused Alisa.

"Yeah, cute, isn't it?" I asked, feeling the sting of estrogen-soaked tears gathering in my eyes. I patted my tummy, "Hello, Raffi."

"I like 'Raffi,'" said Alisa. "'Raphael' can sound a bit poncey."

Alisa speaks her mind and I love her for it, because it's a beautiful mind. We've always delighted in pushing the envelope, joking, sparring, and kibitzing. Nothing is sacred. This day, I chose to forget that.

"Well, what names do *yooou* like?" I sniffed back childishly.

"I like . . . Atticus." Alisa smiled, not detecting the whiff of hormones bubbling over inside me.

"Atticus?! That's beyond poncey! I know, why don't we call him 'Pe-oncey'? Or how about Rock? Bo? Killer?" I was starting to get on an ugly roll.

While remaining hunched over the appetizers, a mutual friend, a mother of two, chimed in. "The surest way to make a pregnant woman cry is to insult her choice of baby names," she proclaimed between mouthfuls of tiny quiches.

Everyone agreed, remembering that I was sensitive. So we switched topics . . . to circumcision.

TO C OR NOT TO C

Like all elements of pregnancy and parenthood, the decision to circumcise your son will elicit unsolicited opinions, much judgment, and heated passions. The reason we were considering it (if we had a boy) did not have to do with cleanliness, or with ensuring that our son would look like his dad. It was purely due to the fact that I was Jewish, raised Jewish, and closely connected to my culture — if not to organized religion and the sexism enshrined therein.

I have a number of progressive Jewish friends who've chosen not to do it. As one put it, "I don't care enough about what my parents think to do this to my child." The problem for me was that I did. If we had a boy and didn't circumcise him, would I be excluding him from his tribe? Confusing his identity? Cutting him off (whoops) from me and a soulful connection to my family? Or would I just be saving him from a painful, bloody welcome to planet earth?

My mother believes that the blood is part of it. There is something visceral and tribal in the entire community standing around in your living room at seven-thirty in the morning, eating bagels, smoked fish, pastries; whispering into each other's ears with coffee breath, crying with you, singing to your child: Welcome to the world of joy, disappointment, pain. Being Jewish ain't a barrel of laughs. Have some rugalach.

Janis decided that this one was up to me. If she had birthed the child and it was a boy, we wouldn't do it. Since the baby would be Jewish by blood, she deferred the decision. There was only one problem. I hate making decisions. I usually get away without having to by pretending that I'm easygoing:

"Oh, I don't care, I'll eat anything."

"Do *you* want me to drive?"

"No, really, I'd see *Love Actually* again, if that's what *you* want."

Underneath this affable exterior is a snake pit of hesitation: what if I make the wrong choice and everyone's unhappy?

So I vacillated. Although it was a private struggle in our household, that did not stop people from weighing in. "How ya feeling? Great. Anyways, listen, if it's a boy, you gonna snip him?" When we said we weren't sure yet, some gay male friends of ours were outraged, mourning the loss of the flap of skin that they never got to know. They were adamant that they could be having more sexual sensation than they were. They asserted that this brutal act was symbolic of a loss of control and choice to which we subject children. I was pretty sure one friend was going to rebirth himself right there in the Starbucks with his foamy latte and the cute Coffee Associates behind the counter as witnesses.

The most offensive comments came from a male friend who suggested it was akin to female genital mutilation (FGM) – the forced removal of a pubescent girl's clitoris and often part of her labia. Women who've endured the torture of FGM, often without anaesthetic, have health problems through their lives and rarely are able to feel any sexual pleasure at all. A better analogy would be the removal of the entire penis.

Then there was my sister, who said, "If you do it, his partners, male or female, will thank you." She was clear that the "helmet," the "aardvark," the "hood" was more trouble than it was worth, got dirty, and wasn't terribly attractive. Other friends simply accepted that it was something that had to be done, like his first blood tests, cutting the chord, or vaccinations (another sensitive and highly politicized topic).

Once we made the decision, we shut up about it. We couldn't bear being forced to justify. Especially when, at the aforementioned brunch, we were asked how we could we think of "chopping" our unborn child, should he be a boy? This casual choice of language was met by stunned silence, tears, and an immature fit of temper – all by me.

I admit I didn't handle moments of conflict well during the pregnancy. I wish I could have engaged in spirited, intelligent debate. Instead, the hormones raged, my face got hot and tight. I was convinced that my very identity was being challenged.

This didn't stop me from eating all their guacamole.

Being a willing member of any faith-based culture can be difficult in an urban modern world. We all recognize the injustices, the blood spilled in the name of religion. But in this case, culture exerted an insistent tidal pull that I had to answer.

CRAVINGS

Speaking of tidal pulls, one day I laid out a proclamation, "Do not let me go grocery shopping alone any more."

In the third trimester, the need to graze intensified. Gone were the ravenous "must eat now or will pass out and/or punch someone in the throat" feelings, but because the baby was now putting so much pressure on my internal organs, I could only eat a little at a time. So I needed to eat more often. And I did.

One of my favourite things to do at this point in the pregnancy was to take a long walk to the grocery store and buy food.

There I was, trolling for bounty at the Loblaws, when I picked up something that I had never purchased in my adult life – liver. Yes, gross, bloody liver.

A voice inside me said, "Pick it up, pick it up, pick it up. Put it in your cart." I tossed it in the cart like a zombie.

Then another voice said, "What are you doing? It's liver. Put it back."

Before I could shift my bulkiness and turn my cart, the first voice reasserted itself, "Do it, eat it, you want it, pick it up pick it up pick it up!"

It only cost $2.59, which I thought was outrageously cheap for some living creature's vital organ. I assured myself that the liver would end up stuck to the side of the freezer with the wontons, veggie chicken fingers, no-name waffles, and stale reefers. So I nonchalantly tossed the bloody organ into my cart with the hummus and the low-fat Pringles.

"And some asparagus –"

"All right already," I shushed.

I got the liver home. I had to call my sister in Missouri to ask her how to cook it. It was mid-afternoon and she was at work.

Apparently, one fries it. In oil. Being an actor and a former fat kid, I habitually tried to avoid the frying and eating of things. Especially the entrails of a formerly living being. Yet here I was ladling the olive oil into the sizzling pan. I added the onions and plopped in the spongy meat. It smelled delicious.

I figured I'd cook it all and then eat it at the dinner hour, like civilized meat-eaters do. But here it was 3:10 in the afternoon, and the liver was cooked, and the voice said, "Dig in."

It was a gorgeous sensation, and a lively, gamy taste. I ate a nice-sized piece, and put the rest in the fridge for a later session of primal carnivorous gorging. Then I took it out and finished it all.

After I wiped the viscera from my chin, I knew there was yet one thing I needed to do. Bake muffins and eat half the mix.

I felt like the baby was ordering room service. "Yes, I'd like some liver fried in onions, some asparagus, and an apple. And if there are any muffins, that would be nice. I'm in Womb 1."

As my friend Rachel, an intuitive writer and observer of social mores, later said, "Liver and muffins? You realize that you are just one step away from cooking your placenta and making us eat it at the bris."

My strongest cravings were for red meat. The bloodier the better. It had been a decade since I had eaten red meat, but in trimester three I was practically a Texan.

Early in my second trimester, Janis and I attended a book launch for a dear friend. The upscale, downtown bar was full of fashionable friends, and waiters carrying flutes of champagne and mini hors d'oeuvres. I followed a gleaming silver tray adorned with tiny nibblies toward the bar. I passed by my dear friend Richard, who was, as usual, eating, with his hands, and his mouth open. Richard can make any food, including fruit salad, look like meat. It's the way he rips at it – obviously relishing it. He is the Jewish version of the King of the Beasts. He was tucking into a steak sandwich as I passed. He called me over to feel my belly and chat. I couldn't hear a word he was saying with the drumming in my ears "steak steak steakidy steak."

I waddled over to the bar, where Janis was shooting the breeze with her highly hip friend Gigi, whom we hadn't seen in ages. I didn't acknowledge their existence. Instead, I ungracefully hoisted myself up on the bar stool, one cheek at a time, and ordered urgently, "One steak sandwich please. Rare. Hurry." Janis stopped in mid-sentence. "Who. Are. You?" she asked haltingly, "and what have you done with my girlfriend?"

A Partial List of Weird and Luscious Cravings

"One time, I insisted that my beleaguered husband drive, at night, all the way downtown to Switzer's Deli and bring back ten knishes. When he returned, I gobbled down all ten! I could barely contain myself. Then I promptly vomited them all up. There was definitely no God that night." – Lily

- My sister craved liverwurst. Laura lives in a small town in the midwestern United States, where there aren't a lot of delis. So she got a friend to *mail* her liverwurst all the way from St. Louis. The deli craving must run in our family.
- Nancy broke fifteen years of vegetarianism to gorge madly on slabs of beef all through her pregnancy.
- Laura also had cravings for V8 vegetable juice (she would drink two litres a day, which I'm sure could not have helped her heartburn).
- Netty craved carbs, especially if they were processed, contained empty calories, and were loaded with food colouring.
- I've heard of women craving salmon, broccoli, and, of course, ice cream and pickles. Yes, together. Even watermelon and celery, which are natural diuretics. However, not many of us crave celery. We're pregnant, not stupid.

A tip for all doting partners and friends of pregnant women: You must respond to all cravings. It is not your partner but the child who is making the request. Your partner is working hard housing something that is shoving her stomach up under her armpits. So don't worry about the nutritional value of a McChicken Sandwich and just get it for her.

Apparently an Indian tradition states that if you don't give in to your cravings when you're pregnant, your child will salivate as a baby. And if you don't know how to cook something that you crave, you must ask someone. They will gladly make it for you because they understand the consequences. They don't want your kid's drool all over their couch.

THE SIZE OF YOU

In one of our prenatal classes at the midwife clinic, we saw a drawing that displayed a cross-section of the internal organs of a pregnant woman as she progresses toward forty weeks. The diagrams looked *exactly* as we felt. Our bladders were indeed flat as pancakes, and our lungs were subletting a bachelor apartment somewhere in our shoulder blades. Our intestines were literally running down our backs, squished so tight that it was a miracle if any of us could poop at all. No wonder we all had heartburn, were panting like old basset hounds, couldn't sleep lying down, and were peeing every twenty minutes.

As I neared the last few months, my belly was becoming as big as the ones that I had seen when I started doing yoga in my second trimester. To my shock, I *was* going to get that big.

I would sit at my desk writing and my belly would literally rest on my thighs. Which is nice because it was a hell of a thing to carry around. My boobs would rest on my stomach, which was nestled on my legs, which were spreading to cover the entire seat.

You may feel undisciplined and unrecognizable at this point. There is, however, a little perk that comes with the weight gain and the bloating: the gigantic tah-tahs. Your boobs will balance out the big booty. The belly will make wherever else you get big look more in perspective. If you can get past the negative messages about fat you may realize that, in fact, you look like a goddess.

Swelling

The size of you in pregnancy is determined by a number of things, not the least of which is genetics. Other factors include: the size of your baby and the accompanying amniotic fluid, the gaining of actual fat to help nourish you and the baby, and . . . water retention.

My midwife explained that the cause of water retention is somewhat a mystery, but that it has to do with cellular osmosis. I stopped listening at this point, because overly scientific explanations – like computer lingo – tend to make me fall asleep. I figured cellular osmosis is yet another example of the baby sucking the life out of you for its own needs.

Nancy had swollen feet long before the rest of us in our midwife prenatal group. They were so puffed up that they shone. Her toes and fingers became numb. Nancy worked in the health-care sector and was always a fount of information. She explained to us gawkers that what she was experiencing was medically termed *edema*, or swelling due to the body's tissues containing an excessive amount of fluid. In her case it was aggravated because she worked in a job where she was on her feet all day, so blood and fluid just lounged about poolside there.

Poor Nancy, we thought. We may be constantly belching, some of us have varicose veins, and one woman's peripheral vision is completely gone, but at least we can put on a pair of pumps.

However, by the end of the midwife classes, tables had turned. Nancy had her beautiful baby daughter and the bones of her toes were materializing. The rest of us had feet the size of clown shoes.

Weight Gain

"You should not gain more than ten to twenty pounds during pregnancy." – Helen MacMurchy, *The Canadian Mother's Book*, 1931

I began the third trimester with what the midwives call "a growth spurt." As a result, I continued to look like a pregnant teen. I was as wide as I was tall and my hair was insanely thick and rebellious, so it had to sit on top of my head in a scrunchy at all times. My maternity clothes of choice were the big shirts, stretchy jeans, running shoes, and jean jackets of the dispossessed youth. No long, cape-y "pregnant real estate lady" looks for me. I tried that and ended up looking like a large toddler playing dress-up in mommy's closet. Neither could I pull off the groovy black tights and furry tight tops that the cool moms wore.

Everyone's weight gain is different, but gain it you will. You need to. Your baby needs you to. There are times when it can be worrying: like if you suddenly start gaining at a much more rapid pace and your sugar and blood pressure are high. Then you might be developing gestational diabetes and also growing a mighty big baby. For most pregnancies, there is no standard of weight gain. Those control freaks who write charts that tell you how much you *should* gain at every stage should check their PalmPilots and see if they might have an opening in their schedules so they can *bite me*! I don't know any two women, or any one woman with more than one pregnancy, who gained weight at the same rate.

Our Amazonian friend Netty put on a mere twenty-five pounds in her whole pregnancy. Not an ounce in the first trimester and then slow and steady all the way through. She also had a very, very fast labour. Five hours. Do not wish her ill.

> "Five hours meant intense slamming contractions and no time for any kind of pain relief. Like jumping out of a plane without a parachute." – Netty

Some women put weight on in little spurts. They plateau for weeks and then have sudden growth. Tammy said to me near the middle of her third trimester, "Pregnancy isn't such a big deal, is it?" Now, granted, she has a high-pain tolerance. She also didn't put much on until the last four or five weeks. Then she packed it on and started getting a fair amount of edema. By the time she was a few days' overdue, perhaps because she hadn't been used to the slow and steady increase in size, she said that she felt like a ship that had run aground. She could barely move. "Why bother?" I responded, "Let the cat come to you."

When I was feeling low during the pregnancy, I usually found bumping into my neighbour, Maria, gave me a lift. She is one of those actors who is so naturally lovely that you wouldn't expect her to also be really smart, funny, and self-deprecating. One hot day toward the end of my third trimester I saw this slip of a tall, sexy woman ambling toward me saying, "You look beautiful, Mama," and I wanted to run. I did not look beautiful to me. I looked like Blimpy from the Popeye cartoons.

I spilled to the poor woman immediately, "I've been trying not to eat a lot. I even feel like I couldn't be eating that much." Yet there I was, almost fifty pounds heavier. Maria saw the tears gathering in my eyes and said, "Honey, I put on seventy-four pounds with my son."

She then told me a story about a friend of hers who ate everything she wanted in her first pregnancy. Just gave herself permission to go wild. She put on fifty-four pounds. Then, with her second pregnancy, she was really disciplined and ate only healthy foods. She put on forty-eight pounds. Maria advised me to relax, enjoy it, revel in it. Big is beautiful.

I agree. Yet, despite those wise words, despite being well versed in the evil repercussions of "the beauty myth"; despite being able to dissect and analyze the inherent misogyny in society's standards for women and especially mothers; despite doing great big belly dances in public, rolling sexy dances in private; despite it all there were times when my self-esteem plummeted.

Thanks for Sharing

One thing that can make the size that you become more difficult to cope with is the tendency of people to share.

"You must be having a girl because your rear end is so big."

"Thanks."

"Anyways, *French Kiss* is due back tomorrow at three p.m."

Janis and I brought the baby's father to one of the prenatal classes at our midwifery clinic. After the class – an evening filled with crucial information and intense bonding – he offered this succinct observation, "Wow, you're the one who's due last, but you're the *biggest!*" I've never let him forget that. If he has, he'll remember it now.

> "Steve and I went to the midwife's near the end of my third trimester. Steve managed to sneak into the bathroom even though there was a large waiting room full of mildly incontinent pregnant ladies. Since there was a scale in the bathroom and we didn't have one at home, he took the opportunity to weigh himself. As I was booking my next appointment, Steve came bursting out of the bathroom and announced, 'Woo hoo! I lost nine pounds!' The whole waiting room of women slowly turned to glare at Steve. As he shrunk to the size of a dust mite, the receptionist asked me, 'Are you going to keep him?'" – Netty

Author Sheila Kitzinger in her article "Nurturing Mothers" says that in the Caribbean, "When the local midwife goes round to the villages, and sees a young woman coming up to her, she says 'You be getting fat' because the nicest thing you could be told is that you might possibly be pregnant."

However, in our repressed North American culture, calling someone "fat" is considered a high insult. During my pregnancy I was called chubby, fatty, fatso, chunky, and enormous. What is wrong with people? Would they refer to an actual overweight person as "fatty"?

"A nurse at work made a point of loudly exclaiming for all to hear about my 'huge' bum, and another nurse then agreed emphatically. The conversation about my posterior went on for a good five minutes. They meant it as a compliment, but it was a little defeating to hear it so baldly." – Nancy

People who said things like, "Are you sure that's all baby?" or "Whacha got in there? A toddler?" were often friends. I tried to remind myself that they were kidding around, perhaps nervously responding to the monumentously huge size of me with a protective patina of humour. I recalled my own panic at yoga upon seeing the big nine-and-a-half-month-pregnant women. I'm sure I said the wrong thing. I do vaguely recall blurting to some poor soul, "How the hell are you gonna get that *out* of there?"

IT'S LIKE A HEAT WAVE

The summer of 2002 settled in with a vengeance. It was the hottest summer in Toronto in decades. Temperatures reached the low forties Celsius.

I'd heard that pregnant women get really pissed off in the heat. I'd been told tales of women snapping at their partners who were valiantly trying to hose and ice them down. I understood. Because you're not just hot. You're trapped. There is nowhere for the heat to go and no relief. I felt like a kiln, a crock pot, a walking radiator.

Fortunately, Janis and I developed some strategies. She hated using air conditioning in the car because of the damage it does to the environment. I needed the air conditioning on high blown directly into my face or I would damage the environment by killing someone. So, our compromise was that she'd angle her vents toward me, and we wouldn't turn it to High. Perfect. Symbiosis.

One of the major disadvantages of being pregnant in the summer is that you have to buy shorts. I tended to get stuck wearing shorts-overalls. This did nothing to dispel the pregnant-teen-runaway look.

Near the end, I gave up all pretense of modesty. I'd nonchalantly wipe the sweat out from under my boobs or the crack of my ass, and just keep on a'walking. . . .

Of course, being in the third trimester in the winter has its joys too. It's harder to get out in the cold and one could get nervous of the snow and ice and end up feeling incredibly trapped. I was at least able to get fresh air, sunshine, and cool water to swim in.

"I slipped on the ice when I was eight months' pregnant. All the people around me panicked, terrified that I might go into labour right in front of them." – Michelle, mother of three

COPING MECHANISMS FOR THE "BIG MAMA"
1) Say these words with me: "I do not bend or run." Tying shoes is also out. It's slip-on adjustable sandals or boots. And put a stool near your front door so you can slide your foot into your shoe at a no-bending-needed height.
2) Collect as many pillows as you can to bolster your belly and boobs for sleeping or long stretches of sitting. Or get one of those body pillows that look like the big lude sausage thing that Ann-Margret rides in The Who's movie *Tommy*.
3) Pamper yourself. I noted that we were getting terribly bourgeois as we anticipated our baby. I joked about wanting to hire an illegal child labourer to walk around with me and hold up my boobs. I insisted we get a dishwasher. If that's out for you, then at least use your partner or friends as Sherpas.

Steve redeemed himself in many ways after his "I lost nine

pounds" debacle. One was by becoming Netty's personal escalator in the last week.

"There is a large hill at the end of a walk that we like to take with our dogs. Steve would get behind me and push me up the last bit. I really should have someone do this for me all the time." – Netty

Luckily for Steve, Netty went into labour early.

4) Tucks. They are a cool cloth that you can use if you get hemorrhoids. 'Nuff said.

5) Robin, mother of twins and the definition of the gallows humorist, had a more radical coping strategy: "My idea of coping was an axe in my head. I thought that would have ended a lot of what I was feeling."

6) Get in the water. With a snorkel. Ruth moved into a new house with a pool during the summer that I was pregnant. I told her not to be alarmed if she came home at night and saw a gigantic pregnant woman floating face up in her backyard. She asked me not to drip on her carpets.

When I was about a week overdue I experienced a true moment of grace. Netty and Steve, following their outdoor-adventure freak impulses, took us to a deserted lake about an hour out of Toronto in an attempt to distract and cool me. I thought they were very brave to tempt fate in this way, so I resisted the urge to pretend to go into labour on the highway.

Netty gave me a mask and a snorkel. Despite looking insane, I went into the water immediately. The snorkel allowed me to keep my neck and head in line with my body. I didn't have to fight gravity and my bulk to get air. My big body was gently rolling in the water, my belly balancing me perfectly. I was at one with the motion of the waves, floating gently, like my baby within me. Bliss.

BIG BABY MOVEMENT

As I got bigger, I used to engage in what we dubbed "Bean-TV," ignoring all other activity that occurred around me and instead watching my naked belly roll and move and buck as the baby seemed to be pushing off the side of the pool. Sometimes half the belly was pressing up, like a whale trying to surface, and the other half looked deflated, like a cake that didn't quite rise.

The midwives warned not to worry if sometimes the movement stops for a bit. The baby needs to sleep too. Every time I got concerned that The Bean wasn't moving, I'd say to my belly, "Come on now, Bean, I need you to move for Mama because I'm Jewish and I'm getting nervous." Invariably, just as panic crept up my chest, The Bean would kick the hell out of me.

Babies seem to get a lot of hiccups. They are taking in amniotic fluid and their little diaphragms are practising contracting to push it out. Some women feel it in their lower backs, a rhythmic tickling. A hard-core rock-vixen friend described it poetically as "butterfly wings."

One night, I was up at about 5 a.m. with lots and lots of head-butting, hiccuping, and all four limbs in a flurry of drumming. Janis woke up and saw that I was awake. I told her to go back to sleep, and she rolled over, put her head on my shoulder as she often does, and then she put her hand and arm on my belly. The baby stopped. It just calmed down. And so did I.

INSOMNIA

"By the way, as far as the 3 a.m. awakenings – I guess that is your subconscious getting you prepared! I would take that opportunity to put on some beautiful, soothing meditative-type music, have a cup of raspberry-leaf tea with honey, and start imagining My Child's Perfect Life, down to the last detail, with absolutely *no* references to 'that couldn't happen because. . . .' You have to describe it exactly or your fairy-godmother won't know what to create for you!" – Jamie, mother of one

Insomnia is partly due to physical discomfort. Sleeping flat on your back becomes much harder now. If I didn't sleep sitting upright, in a position that would force the baby's head farther down my pelvis and give my lungs more room, I couldn't breathe. I felt like I was suffocating. So I slept in a reclining L shape.

"I could not sleep in a regular bed for more then one hour. I had to move to a waterbed because my own weight was causing my hips a lot of pain. What a trip it was. I know I want another baby, so I will have to go through this again. Luckily it was worth it." – Laura

The leg cramps may come in earnest now. Getting out of bed without mechanical assistance to do the leg-cramp dance would be tragic if it weren't so cartoony. There you are, naked, sweating, heaving yourself around your bedroom floor with one foot flexed within an inch of its life, desperately trying to stretch out that calf. You will probably be swearing a little too. Forgive your partner for the giggles that will escape as they try to come up with something helpful to do.

Then there's the psychological pressure. Knowing that your life will change irrevocably. Knowing labour is coming. My brain wouldn't let me sleep, as I recounted in an early-morning e-mail to a friend, "I've been up since 2:30 a.m. This is the most extreme one yet. I am UP UP UP! SO awake. I had some warm milk, so maybe I'll sleep. I've been thinking about the drive to the hospital in labour, about the labour itself, arriving at the hospital and how will I get upstairs to the room. What I will wear . . . By the way, hot milk is GROSS!"

Although I was struggling to finish a project by my due date and had just started a new one, I occasionally felt like the world was passing me by. I obsessed that I not only had few irons, but that my fire had fizzled out.

So I took the opportunity that my insomnia provided to read scary books about labour in the middle of the night. I read them with the intention of allowing both Janis and I to become familiar with what was to come. Instead, they freaked the hell out of me, made me worry that we weren't doing enough to prepare, and kept me awake even more.

Although insomnia can generally be attributed to all of the above factors, there is also a *unique* wakefulness that occurs. Many parents told me that it was my body practising for motherhood. I asked why my body couldn't just rest up at night and practise during the day.

BRAXTON HICKS

You may also have mild practice contractions, called Braxton Hicks after the doctor who "discovered" them. It can feel like odd little squeezes, like someone is putting a lot of pressure on your belly. Some women find them completely inoffensive, and others experience a lot of discomfort. They can get more intense and frequent while you're walking. Every so often you may have to stop and loudly say "Oy," even if you're not Jewish.

My midwives explained that the uterus is "tuning up" for labour. It is sending signals to the muscles that comprise it to contract. The muscles of the uterus of a pregnant woman become the largest and strongest muscle group in the body. It's so big that it doesn't communicate properly. Like the federal government. The left wing isn't quite in synch with the centre. And the right wing is completely out to lunch. Consequently, parts of the muscle practise contracting at different times. In labour the whole team comes together and squeezes the hell out of you, dilates that cervix, and gets that baby *out*.

When these Braxton Hicks occur while you're sleeping, they may wake you. While you're up, you might as well go pee. Since someone really should install a winch and crane to help you to get out of bed, and no one has yet, it may take a lot of effort to get up on your own. Once you do get up and waddle down the hall to the loo, manage to lower that bulk onto the toilet, pee, and somehow wipe, possibly from the back, getting yourself back into bed without said crane is much too arduous. So that cute little practice contraction has just awakened you for the next hour or three.

Since you're up, you might as well go make a list of things you want for your baby shower.

GETTING THE ROOM READY – THE BABY SHOWER

Some energetic, generous friends of ours offered to hold a baby shower for us. It became a community event. I was one of the few in my immediate circle to be pregnant at the time. Also, Janis and I didn't have a wedding or a commitment ceremony so it was a way of celebrating our relationship. At that point we'd been together seven years. Due to the intense nature of two women as partners, lesbian years are a bit like dog years, so our seven years might be more equivalent to seventeen in a straight relationship.

My mother doesn't believe in showers before the baby comes. Part of that Jewish superstition of "God forbid you should celebrate something good before it actually happens and then almost wish a bad thing to happen instead – what are you crazy, tempting fate?! Why don't you just go bang yourself in the head with something?!"

But one thing my mother *loves* to do, as this e-mail illustrates, is make lists:

"So, I was figuring the following:

Regarding the colour of the dresser for the new beautiful wonderful baby (*k'nein a hora*). We'd like it to match the colour of the crib and chair that your friends Leah and Leslie already gave you. It seems that colours are in style during certain years, just like with clothing and upholstery and paint. There are I figure three solutions: 1) you ask the people who gave you the chair and/or the crib for the name of the colour of the wood. 2) is it okay, if we cannot get the exact same colour to get a light wooden dresser? 3) we replace the crib and chair with something that matches the dresser we're getting you. What do you think?"

These e-mails came fast and furious, getting more detailed every day. For someone who claimed she didn't want to think about shopping until after the baby arrived, who wrestled with the "evil eye" daily, who embraced the healthy wariness of five thousand years of history, the woman was obsessed with lists.

So between her and our research of books and other parents, we came up with a partial inventory (the parentheses are mine).

Maybe this will be helpful for you and allow you to spend your last few weeks as a singular being thinking of more important things – like reorganizing your kitchen cupboards.

The Bean's Shower List
- crib
- change table
- gliding rocking chair – they have ones that recline so Mama can sleep too
- car seat
- a swing
- receiving blankets
- newborn clothes and diapers

- clothes and diapers for LATER
- diaper pail
- diaper bag
- bathtub for baby (we *do* have our own and I *have* been living in it)
- bottles and nipples (yoiks)
- newborn baby toys and mobiles (okay, I'm freaking myself out)
- baby creams for diaper rash and whatever baby's need creams for
- sling for carrying baby like a monkey
- a monkey
- sleepers
- nasal aspirator (you have GOT to be kidding)!

As the reality of what was happening inside me made itself more evident, besides lists, I sunk into some primal terrors. I immediately took them out on Janis.

THE WALKMAN

I had started going for long walks in the morning. Mostly because I still could. I would start by walking Janis and her bike across the park, after which she would ride off to her job. One morning when we said our usual goodbyes at the corner, I realized that she was about to get on her bike with her Walkman on. I asked her to take it off.

"It's not safe," I heard myself burble, "you won't be able to hear oncoming traffic."

"I've done it a million times. I'll put the volume on low," Janis said and tried to kiss me goodbye. I was not having any of it. I was furious that she would put herself at risk in front of me, with the baby coming. I began grabbing for the Walkman.

"Gimme that!" I swung at her helmet with my swollen paw.

"Diane!" Janis was shocked.

"Gimme that NOW!"

"Stop it. You can't crush *my* dreams out of *your* fear," Janis warned, trying to de-escalate us both using logic. Didn't work.

"This isn't some big-deal dream like skydiving or rock climbing," I gesticulated wildly. "You want to do that, sure. After the baby. I'll spot you. But this is just stupid!"

"Is this how you're going to be from now on?"

"I don't know!" I shouted, "I'VE NEVER BEEN PREGNANT BEFORE."

I walked away in a rage. I surreptitiously glanced back a few times and saw Janis following me. The last time I tried to sneak a peak, she held my gaze, her hands on her hips. I tore my eyes away from her and kept walking. It was the first time in seven years that we walked away mad.

This, of course, terrified me even more. Now, she'd bike with the Walkman on, get hit by a car, and the last moment we had together would be a fight.

I shook the whole way home, where, following the nudgy voice of my ancestors, I reasoned that the problem was that we were *too* happy. Maybe the universe might want to end our joy? Creating life makes you realize how easy it would be to have it snuffed out in an instant.

I wasn't able to articulate this to Janis in the moment. All I knew was that this was one of those times in our relationship when I wanted to kick and scream against the one who loved me most. When I wanted special allowances to play the pregnancy card. And I wanted not to have to ask for it.

Here's some free advice for partners: Now is not the time to buy a motorcycle. I know that you have a wild impulse to do so. You may be feeling frightened that this child is going to limit your lifestyle. It will. But it's time to grow up.

Eventually Janis and I came to the same place and accepted this responsibility. I just got there faster because I was the one who was stuffed to the gills with baby.

PHYSICAL VULNERABILITY

As I got bigger and my limbs got looser, I felt a kind of physical vulnerability that I hadn't experienced since I was a teenager. Back then, I used to be terribly fearful. My instinct was not "fight or flight" but "pass out or puke."

Like many women, I tended to deal with my anger by hyperventilating, bursting into tears, and sulking. I was even worse at managing fear. Which is why I got into boxing.

You may ask, What would prompt an otherwise sensible, university-educated, thirty-something woman to step into a rancid-smelling gym, don sweat-soaked headgear, and get punched in the eye? If you had asked me that question a few years ago I would have said, "Nothing on earth" or "$40,000," depending on the day.

Some questions I was frequently asked when I mentioned my boxing obsession were: "Why don't you do something else to get in shape?" "What if you get hurt?" and "You pay for this?!" My usual answer was, "Mom, please, I like it."

The intense boxing training that I engaged in before the pregnancy certainly got me into good shape. I also developed fearlessness, and a gleeful road rage.

A month before I got pregnant, I parked my car on the side of the road, on the way to do some errands. I got out and, with a plastic bag of garbage in my hand, was waiting for traffic to clear so I could cross the street. A young man in a low-slung, sporty-but-you-know-Daddy-bought-it car slid partially into the right lane, dangerously close to me. As he passed me, for no reason at all, he honked. It startled me and without thinking I smashed my bag of garbage down hard on the hood of his car.

The next thing I knew, he screeched to a stop in front of me. He got out of his car, leaving a gum-chewing woman in the passenger seat – watching with ennui through the side mirror. He stormed toward me. Much to his surprise, I stormed toward him. He yelled that I had frightened his girlfriend.

"Fuck your girlfriend and fuck you," I growled as I sized him up. He was maybe five inches taller than me, soft around the middle, little goatee, wraparound sunglasses. He pounded his fist on the roof of my car and said, "If you weren't a woman I'd . . ."

I sidled right up to him, my nose at his chin, and said slowly and deliberately, "I am not afraid of you." I wasn't. I could clearly imagine what I'd do. Duck his punch, then uppercut to the chin, two hooks to the ribs, jab jab to the head, slip, and I'm out of there. My fists were clenched, my muscles taut in anticipation. I knew that I wouldn't throw the first punch, so I pushed us both as close as possible to the line at which he would snap.

He paused and walked back to his car, giving my bumper a face-saving final kick. For the first time in my life, I was not afraid. Calm inwardly and coiled outwardly.

Eight months later, I had changed from that strutting pugilist into a person who was afraid to walk on the ice in case she would slip; who couldn't canter up a hill without getting winded; who needed a mechanism to untie her shoes. More than that, I *felt* terribly vulnerable. If someone wanted to hurt me, I couldn't put up much of a fight. If I was bumped, I'd fall. All I could think about was my supreme responsibility: the care and nurturing of this being who needed to come through me into the world. I *couldn't* fall.

Years of hard physical and psychological work seemed to be for naught. I became something that I hadn't been in years: cautious.

THE HOME STRE-E-E-ETCH

The last week before giving birth is "the great leveller" of pregnancies. No matter how the past thirty-nine weeks went for you – miserable or joyous – this will undoubtably be a test.

Do not curse yourself if you said, "Pregnancy's a breeze" at week thirty-eight. You are not being punished. This is simply nature's way of making you want, plead, and beg to go into labour.

Expecting this, perhaps your last week won't feel so bad. This is what happened to me. I read in every book how nasty I would become, how uncomfortable and sore. I anticipated hell on earth, so when it came, it didn't seem that bad. Like when you read terrible reviews of a movie, and when you see it you say, "I kinda liked *Daddy Day Care*."

People refer to women in their ninth month with the prefix "poor," as in "Poor Vickie can't get around the counter" or "Poor Aisha can barely move." I'm sure people said of me, "Poor Diane, she looks like a cross between Animal from *The Muppet Show* and Andy Rooney."

I saw a picture of my mom when she was abundantly pregnant with me in the late 1960s. She was radiant. She stood demurely, her legs crossed at the ankle. She wore a blousie maternity dress with the appropriate empire waist, and a knowing smile. Her hair was piled on top of her head in stiff waves, like a wedding cake. Her dress fell perfectly over her burgeoning belly, giving her a warm hug. She glowed with satisfied fecundity.

I also have a picture of me at the end of my ninth month. In my plaid, supersized husky-boy shirt and my huge old-man shorts – the kind with extra room for the saggy sack. I looked like a short, fat guy with a beer gut. And I acted like one too. I had gas, heartburn, trouble breathing and bending. I was impatient, irritable, and I sat with my feet up like I had gout.

To make matters more alarming, I gained almost five pounds in the six days before my due date. This made me feel completely mystified, morose, and monstrous. I was also experiencing lots of cramps, Braxton Hicks, and weepiness.

So I watched *Oprah*. It was one of those shows where she gives away tons of crap. "Why can't *I* have a compact serviette folder?" I wailed to the cosmos. "How will I ever cope with a baby when I have no pen-that-takes-pictures?!"

Somewhere between tiny wristwatches that remind you to call your mother and fishcake-makers, I fell asleep. In a position that shoved my lungs up my nose. I woke up choking and coughing, which led to peeing in my pants and then "running" up the stairs trying to catch the pee before another cough came. I didn't make it.

In the meantime, my sweetie had come home and was on the phone. She didn't immediately get off to see if this galumphing, panting, swearing, leaking being was all right. This incensed me. I attacked.

"Who the *hell* was on the phone?!"

"My dad."

"What the *hell* did he want?!"

"To see how you were feeling."

Flummoxed, I fished for things to be mad at her for. Why wasn't she reading the grotesque labour literature that I left for her? She didn't want to do perineal massage. She wouldn't help me with my Kegel exercises. She didn't want to review our baby shower lists. Did she even know the stages of labour? Their length, duration, and intensity? Had she purchased raspberry tea or gigantic Kotexy blue pads for when my water breaks?

"Am I alone here?!" I collapsed onto the bed, causing it to skid eight inches from the wall.

Thinking quickly, she responded to my accusations by asking me to explain where all this angst originated. I replied with the sanity of a hyena that because of watching *Oprah* I coughed, choked, and peed. Even I couldn't help but laugh.

I now understand that most partners simply can't be as "under your skin" as you and the baby are. There's no point in testing them. They will fail.

Also, they're probably doing many sweet and kind things for you and the baby every day. Unbeknownst to me, my partner had met with a sommelier so she could buy me a special bottle of wine to enjoy in pre-labour. This was a treat the midwives suggested for really early labour, to loosen you up. Since I hadn't imbibed in nine months, she blew a bundle. She also bought lovely champagne for after the birth. We didn't end up drinking it then, but we did crack it open on his first birthday and got wonderfully hammered together.

BYE-BYE DUE DATE

I was uncomfortable enough in the week before my due date that I assumed I would be going into labour early. The midwives were noncommittal, though they did tell me that the baby was turned with its back facing me – called posterior – which could result in painful back-labour. They assured me that I shouldn't worry because The Bean could still turn. They also said that my cervix was not yet soft and was facing posterior. It needed to drop forward and thin out (or "efface") to signal that labour was about to begin.

Since the midwives didn't tell me what I wanted to hear (that this pregnancy would be over any day now), I sought out other people's advice. So, about a day or two from my due date, I found myself hovering around the older mothers (and the dessert table) at my friend Kate's fiftieth birthday party.

With cheekfuls of chocolate mousse, I got into an officially deep conversation with a mother of three whom I barely knew. She gazed intently into my eyes, telling me that we were about to become sisters in the most amazing vocation the universe can offer. That the joy was certain to be miraculous. I was trying to relax, listen, and display inner-mama peace to her. I failed, as I tend to find conversations where people unblinkingly look me in the eye fidget-inducing.

She ignored my schoolgirl twitchiness and informed me that mothers always "know" if they will be having a boy or a girl, and when they will go into labour. One just has to focus, find a calm place, mentally go "inside" your mind, and ask. The answer will come. I came up with "girl" and "early."

By a day before my due date, the Braxton Hicks had eased and the cramps were less frequent, which was not making me happy, because I was hoping the previous week's discomfort was building to labour.

Instead, I got a reprieve. The baby's head had dropped quite a bit, so I could finally breath. I slept more with less interruptions for cramps or Braxton Hicks. The great Toronto heat wave broke for a day or two. I felt good, spry, sexy. I paraded about with the belly exposed for all to see, knowing that soon it would be over.

I even felt like having sex. Janis was swamped at work, but was being so considerate of me. Plus, she always told me I looked beautiful. Out of clothes, she was right. The boldness of the breasts and booty and the vivid tumultuousness of the stomach made for an image of striking and powerful splendour.

Hopefully you will be granted a moment or two in the oasis that I stumbled into near the end. If so, please note the following:

Sex Positions for Nine Months

- *Prone*: Not good, can't breath, bad heartburn, acid reflux, and baby's movements are obvious and unnerving.
- *Sitting Straight Up*: It's almost impossible to find or access anything from there. Yet I have friends that actually could have sex this way. The pregnant woman was propped up on pillows so that her back was supported. I was way way way too huge for this.

- *Doggy Style*: The second most popular choice among moms I spoke with. It's okay for a bit, then you get heartburn – gotta stop for a Tums. Also, the pressure on the back can be a bit much.
- *Sideways*: The most popular choice: lying sideways with the pregnant partner in front. It was described as "the scissor position."

I wasn't the only one intrigued by the challenge of home-stretch sex. My pals weighed in too.

"Okay, let me think back. Sex, what is that? Oh yeah. I would say the position for us gals that were big, no I mean, really big mamas, would be a scissor-like position from behind. Does that make any sense? I will give more details over the phone if you need. It will cost $2.99 each minute." – Victoria, mother of one

Netty said that her husband was willing for her to pass on this information to me, as long as I told him in great detail what it was *exactly* that Janis and I do in bed. . . .

"As for the sex questions, this makes me laugh. The reality is that as you get bigger and bigger there is not much you can actually do to get laid. I must admit that sex was also one of the last things on my mind when I was the size of a hippo trying to move. My huge, bloated Hobbit tootsies did not help either. Let's just say that I can count on one hand the number of times we had sex in the second and third trimesters combined." – Elizabeth, mother of one

It is quite common for a woman in the late stages of pregnancy to find sex physically awkward and difficult. Elizabeth has a caring partner who came up with a great idea that I'll pass on to all of you. If you are a demure flower and get red-faced easily, I apologize. But I know you want to read on.

> "My husband knew how frustrating all this was for me. So he got me a very interesting Valentine's gift. He went into the local sex shop and explained to the guy behind the counter what was happening. The guy recommended a dildo. This dildo was a curved wand with a ball on the end. It was a fantastic gift because the curved wand allowed me to get around my belly with it. I know this sounds funny, but at least I had that to play with."

The most common difficulty with sex in the later trimesters that I've heard came from the partners. Many of them simply could not go there mentally. They just could not do it thinking of their little baby in there. They keep worrying that the baby might get scared from all the bumping.

So with all these factors, sex was not such an option for us. We assured each other that we'd get back to it after the baby . . . WRONG.

PRE-BIRTH CALISTHENICS FOR THE OVERACHIEVER

To keep busy, I read up on labour. I flipped to the section on pain-management techniques in the book *The Birth Partner* by Penny Simkin. She suggested that in order to learn to cope with the intense pain that is coming, you hold an ice cube in your hand very tightly for a minute at a time. In that minute, you practise methods of dealing with pain, from distracting yourself to going "into" the pain. You get your partner to do it too so that you both can share in the discovery. Unfortunately, you can't share labour pain with them.

I found this a good exercise, and I even remembered some of it in early labour, but it became completely irrelevant when active labour actually hit. At that point, Janis and I could have had ice cubes up our *noses* and we would have not been aware of them.

The other exercise that is suggested is the perineal massage. The perineum is the area of muscle and nerves that forms a figure eight around your tushie and hoochee. During birth, the perineal tissue stretches to let the baby's head out. Some people suggest that massaging that area with oil, or stretching it before labour, helps to avoid tearing. They suggest you get your partner to insert their thumbs into your vagina and stretch it outward in a circular motion. You will feel a burning sensation, a precursor to the "ring of fire" that occurs when the baby's big old head is sitting there, stuck in your hoo-haw waiting to be pushed out. It was interesting to get a sense of what it all might feel like. Although, I have to admit we got lazy. Plus I had the baby's room to paint.

> "Steve asked me if I wanted him to stick his big wood-worker hands in there to do a little perineal stretch. I asked him if he would like me to stretch his anus." – Netty

An image from the book *Birthing from Within* by Pam England and Rob Horowitz equated women who were about to enter childbirth to soldiers in battle. They referred to them as warriors who needed courage. I liked that image of myself and what I was about to do much more than that of the earth-embracing, red-tent entering, tub-birthing mother-goddess. Or than the other extreme: the epidural-at-once, faxing-in-the-labour-room, get-the-night nurse, too-posh-to-push "modern" mom. Childbirth is a bloody, challenging, dangerous enterprise, and once you start you have no choice but to follow your body's commands. Lock 'n' load, warrior women!

HORROR STORIES FROM OUR MOTHERS

My partner, my son, and I are living in a great city at a great time. We have access to midwives and doctors. We can have our babies in hospitals and/or at home. We can read a variety of books and take classes. Our partners are encouraged to be an integral part of the process. We do not have to go through labour and childbirth alone.

Our mothers were not so lucky. While we got to make a "birth plan," many women of our mothers' generation were not given much choice as to how they gave birth, or with whom.

"I found labouring to be a solitary experience. . . . My husband's role in the whole birthing process was to spray my stitches for a few days after I got home. I thought he would pass out the first time he set eyes on his target." – Ruthy, mother of David, bubbe (grandmother) of Eli

In one of the most extreme versions of the system controlling the women it was supposed to serve, Ruthy describes how her wrists were strapped down so they could get an ether mask on her.

"I started shaking my head 'no.' My tormentor at the head of the table didn't care. He had a job to do and, by Jove, he was going to do it. It was at this point that I figured out why my hands had been tied down . . . to keep me from hitting the jerk. I eventually fought him off and my baby arrived with me conscious. I figured that delivery couldn't be any worse than labour and no one had offered me gas then."

Far from being konked out, my needs and well-being were actively solicited. My mother, Lily, described how she was given drugs and came in and out of consciousness to hear someone moaning and screaming, and realized that it was her.

"I was told to be quiet and that I'd get over it. The baby was born and immediately whisked away. I came to consciousness hours later. A nurse arrived and I asked what happened. The nurse said, 'You'll have to start all over again.' I gasped in terror.

The nurse quickly explained that she meant that now that I had *had* a baby, I'd have to start all over again on another one. I replied that my husband would be having the next one."

While potential complications during delivery were explained to me in graphic detail, women of Janis's mother's generation were deliberately kept in the dark.

"A friend recently told me how she was labouring away for hours with a baby that was breech. The doctor kept encouraging her to try to push him out, which, with a breech baby, could be a difficult, painful, and sometimes dangerous thing to do. It was so painful that my friend held back a bit on the pushing. She had no idea that time was of the essence because *no one had informed her that her baby was breech!* Her husband, cooling his heals in the waiting room, knew. Her mother knew. The doctor decided not to tell the woman who was actually having the baby." – Doris, mother of three, grandmother of Eli

Once our son arrived, we got to keep him in the hospital room with us and were given lots of help with breastfeeding. Our mothers' babies were taken from them after birth and brought back every four hours for scheduled feedings. Often breastfeeding was not encouraged or explained. Doris had no choice about breast or bottle. Her babies were simply taken and given formula.

Lily recalled two very vivid images that highlight how far we've come:

"There was a stretcher in the hallway. A young girl was lying there, on her side, fully pregnant and in obvious agony. She stayed motionless and silent. No one was with her. I asked the nurse who this girl was. The nurse replied, dismissively. 'Oh don't worry about her. She's not married.' . . ."

". . . The Case Room was small; there were two hospital beds. One woman was already on one of the beds. I couldn't see her, but I could hear her screaming and moaning by turns. When I tried to look in her direction, I was told, 'Don't worry about her, she's Italian. They all scream.' I was to learn later that she died."

The one thing that both Lily and Doris appreciated from their day was that they were able to stay in hospital longer than mothers generally do now. My mother said that if you had a boy you stayed for eight days – to get the circumcision done (no agonizing over that decision) – and for girls you stayed for five. We wish we had stayed longer, to get sleep, more help with breastfeeding, and to limit the number and length of visits.

There is much yet to fight for. We need to be reminded of how far we've come and that the battles we fight now are part of that continuum. We do *not* want to go back there. As my mother concludes, "So, I guess the gist of this is that we did not know much and relied on experts to help us. And they failed us. And we knew it was wrong. And we kept talking about it and doing research so that this misery would end with our generation."

Let's hope our daughters and sons have it even better than we do now.

— • • —

A tip. Mothers advised me, and I will advise you, to take time alone. Go to a café, eat a Caesar salad, and read a book. Make spontaneous dates with friends. And spend time with your partner. You will have trouble finding it very soon.

— • • —

6
So That's Why It's Called "Labour"

It was simply the most intense pain I've ever endured. Granted I've never had a piece of glass fly into my eye or an ex tell me that I was the worst lover they've ever had. I have experienced some physical pain, though, and nothing felt like this.

I got together with a group of moms from prenatal yoga one evening almost a year after my son was born. With wine and without our babies. We immediately, guiltily, thirstily started whispering our labour stories like drug addicts at an NA meeting. We were spilling our battle exploits, trying to best one another with dreadful or miraculous details, until someone relayed the tale of a woman in a remote village in Mexico who performed a C-section on herself with a kitchen knife. That kind of topped 'em all. As my friend Bruce says, "I've noticed that women tell their birth stories like old men tell their war stories, 'I was at Vimy Ridge when my water broke! . . .'"

This urge to share can be so overwhelming that it can lead you to the wrong people, at the wrong time. Like still-pregnant women who ask an innocent question like, "Is labour pain like menstrual cramps?" Yeah, times a *thousand*! Yeah, if you happen to be menstruating while an *elephant stands on your lap*! Yeah, if you were menstruating *chainsaws*!

I should have known better because I was one of those need-to-know-nerds who, as I neared week forty-two of the forty-week gestation period, was compelled to ask all the moms I met what labour felt like, thinking foolishly that that information would help me to prepare. The following are some of the ways it was described to me:

- a spiralling ripping sort of pain
- a herniated vertebrae, but all over your body
- "I can't tell you. No, actually, I won't tell you."
- a beautiful, joyful opening sensation

The midwives said that it was different for every woman, and that it would progress from manageable pain to pain that felt unmanageable, but that I *could* cope and *would* cope. Also, I could have an epidural if I wanted it. My midwife told me that my concern about the "shame" of asking for an epidural was my own issue. They had no judgment around it.

One of the women in our midwife prenatal group was very open from early on that she intended to have as many drugs as possible. In fact, at her eight-month mark, she said that she'd like to start having drugs now and keep at it until her child was old enough to buy them for her. She was not interested in experiencing any more pain. She'd gone through invasive measures to get pregnant, and her resulting pregnancy had been brutal. She'd suffered enough.

Like many women, I dreaded that I would panic, lose my dignity, lose control, not be able to cope with the pain. My biggest fear was that I would be mean to my wonderful partner. That I'd reveal some horrible "real" inner me.

"It was early labour and I was pacing the halls. I would wave at another woman in early labour as we passed each other, both of us in our runners, doing our strong woman thing. Eventually, the other woman went into hard labour. I could hear her moaning all the way down the hall. At one point, I heard the woman's husband say, 'You're doing really well, honey. You're doing so well.' And she yelled back, 'I am not fucking doing well, you fucking asshole!'" – Bev, writer/actor and mother of two

I told my midwife, Sara, this story, pretending I thought it was hilarious. She looked at me calmly and assured me, "You won't do that. You just won't."

START YOUR ESTRO-ENGINES!

My sister and I concur that Mama Nature makes many first mothers late so that they will do ridiculous things in order to go into labour.

The day before my labour began, I was sitting in the heat watching Janis's team play a soccer game (Janis was in Montreal – more on *that* later). I was the team's mascot. Sitting in my tiny lawn chair with my Gatorade and my huge naked belly, I looked like one of those kitschy lawn statues of a smiling bullfrog with sunglasses.

By that time, I was over a week late, and I could see that many of the soccer women were not so much enchanted by me as alarmed. There is something cataclysmic about a hugely pregnant woman in a heat wave. In boxer shorts. And a gigantic sports bra. Belching rhythmically. It unnerves people.

In order for me to deal with their obvious anxiety, and their unhelpful observations like: "Haven't you had that thing yet? . . . It's going to be huge!" I gathered the team and told them that I needed their help. I vowed to the field full of athletic, dewy, young women that I would go into labour and end their terrified anticipation – if they all took their tops off.

Even gigantic, overheated mamas with acid reflux, constipation, and triple chins have a libido. The delightful end of this story is that they did, and I went into labour the next night. So, I suggest you try this method – substituting topless men if that is your predilection.

My sister, Laura, was thirteen days late. In the summer. In Missouri. It wasn't pretty. Granted, the forty-week timeline for pregnancy term is an average. Forty-two weeks falls within a normal range, but it sure didn't feel normal to Laura and me.

Laura went for daily acupuncture on her calves. Apparently the calf is on the energy line to the uterus. I accompanied her one day, expecting to be ushered into a dark, womblike cubby hole of an office, where a stooped, crinkly Asian man would glow with magical possibilities. Instead, we drove her pickup truck to the back of a suburban bungalow. Inside were burnished walnut desks in spacious offices with spotless massage tables, each equipped with discreet electrical gadgets that looked like mauve battery chargers. These "chargers" were attached to a few dozen tiny needles stuck into Laura's puffy shins. Electrical impulses urged her legs to tell her womb to begin getting this kid *out*! Her acupuncturist was a clean-cut, preppy guy who prattled on about his kids and his golf game. He promised her this would work and that she better get ready to go into labour in her truck, ha ha.

She didn't, ho ho.

Some idiot suggested to Laura that she jog. Did I mention her breasts *started off* at triple E? I suggested that the idiot tie an anvil to his waist, get in a sauna, and sprint. See how that feels.

Mary took red and blue cohosh drops and drank raspberry tea. She was also advised to try castor oil. Let me officially warn you: No matter how strongly someone suggests it, DO NOT TRY CASTOR OIL. The principle is that when one has dramatic, unrelenting, furious diarrhea for a length of time, the contractions around the intestines and sphincter can trigger labour. Just what I want: to shit my brains out and then get contractions – or better yet, do both at the same time. The other minor problem with castor oil is that in the case of my few friends who tried it, it didn't work. They were really cleaned out for labour though, and never had to poo the whole time. So that is some consolation. Not enough in my books, but you decide.

Another common method of starting labour is the "stretch and sweep." The midwife or doctor puts a finger or fingers into your tightly clenched, stubborn little cervix and stretches it. Not only does this open it a titch, but it also stimulates the secretion of prostaglandin, the hormone that gets labour started. The stretch and sweeps do give you a taste of the unique way that labour feels in the body. They can also begin the release of "bloody show" – blood and mucus from the cervix. Janis and I could only shout the ridiculous-sounding words *bloody show!* at the top of our lungs, in a pompous British accent. As if announcing the arrival of royalty at a ball, which, in a way, we were.

The other way to get prostaglandins close to the cervix is to have sex. Prostaglandins hang out naturally in semen. Richard said he and his wife were young, horny, and doing it right to the bitter end – in an attempt to get the ball rolling. *I* think he is so old now that his memory is going. It's sad, but at least Richard has three wonderful children to visit him when he goes into "the home."

Usually by a week to ten days past the due date, you will be advised to get an ultrasound to make sure there is still enough amniotic fluid, that your placenta is still vibrant (they do have a shelf life), and to check on the position of the baby. In Toronto, you have to get some sort of intervention by the second week.

We were given a list of the medically assisted methods to induce labour:

- **The insertion of prostaglandin gel directly onto the cervix.** This must be done in hospital, by some yahoo you've never met. You are often asked to wait around for about six hours to see if there has been any effect. Sounds fun. Bring the Yahtzee.
- **Breaking the waters.** No, it's not done with a pin while you lie on a rubber sheet. It's done with a knitting needle while you sit on a potty. (Kidding! This *is* the twenty-first century. No one knits any more.)
- **An IV of oxytocin in what is called a picotin drip.** There is nothing drippy about this. Women who've had it compare it to going from zero to a hundred in a race car. Without seatbelts.

These last two methods tend to "slam" a woman into really hard contractions, and are therefore often accompanied by the epidural. The words *slam* and *contractions* do not need to exist in the same sentence, do they? Yikes.

My midwife said that she was never comfortable predicting things, but from her experience, women will go into labour the night before they are scheduled to be induced.

I made a plan that on the tenth day after my due date, if I hadn't gone into labour on my own, I would go into the hospital for the prostaglandin gel. Although the midwives were happy to wait the full two weeks before they'd have to induce me, I had had enough. To complicate matters, Janis was in Montreal for a week finishing a masters program.

On Janis's third day there, I woke up at 4 a.m. feeling "not right." I never had the "bake chocolate cookies, vacuum the house within an inch of its life, scrub the light sockets" kind of nesting urge. But I felt off. So I called Janis in Montreal, woke her up, and proceeded to scare the crap out of her. She informed me that due to a few frightening conversations she had had with some of the mothers in her program (who all happened to have very fast labours), she'd already booked her ticket to come home the next morning. Would I be okay? I had no idea. Although there was some comfort in knowing someone else was now sleepless and freaking out too.

Labour didn't start that morning. I woke up feeling totally normal. As normal as you can when you're carrying fifty pounds of baby in the worst heat wave in Toronto since 1907.

At midnight that night, the day after the soccer game boob exposures, the day my partner came home, the day before I was scheduled to be induced in hospital, it began.

LABOUR – THE END . . . AND THE BEGINNING

Labour is divided into three stages, preceded by pre-labour – which isn't given its own stage, although it can be a bit of a spot-light hog.

1) Early labour, active labour, and transition make up the first stage.
2) The pushing stage follows.
3) The birth of the placenta is the final stage.

The stages can cascade into one another, but all have distinctive characteristics. I studied every detail about them like the Hebrew-school nerd that I am. I tried to understand and memorize them, as if this was material for an exam, and if I only studied hard enough, I would pass with flying colours, no panic, and little pain.

Pre-labour

Pre-labour is characterized by contractions that come semi-regularly (every thirty minutes or so) but never get stronger, more regular, or closer together. So you can endure, as my sister and Netty did, a number of sleepless nights of icky cramps with not much to show for it.

In Netty's case, the pre-labour did do some work on opening her cervix because once her labour started, a week early, it lasted a shockingly swift five and a half hours. Not long enough to get an epidural. I'm sure it felt like an eternity.

"We were caught in traffic on the way to the hospital, with the baby's head starting to crown. We spent twenty minutes in hospital before Parker was born. The pain was claustro-phobic. I felt like I was trapped in a cave with it. I couldn't fathom that there was really no way out, that no one was going to come and fix it." – Netty

What a shocking betrayal. Someone usually helps: mom, your partner, God. Not now. Now it's down to you.

STAGE ONE
Early Labour
The contractions in early labour last thirty to forty-five seconds, and they can vary from five to twenty minutes apart. They are not as intense or painful as the ones to come in active labour, but how are you to know that while you're in them? In this stage, the cervix dilates from zero to four centimetres.

Unlike on sitcoms, labour doesn't necessarily begin with a big sploosh of waters breaking. They can break anytime before, during, or near the end of labour. Mine sort of leaked out all the way through, and looked pretty clear. We were told that if they were brown or green or had a bad smell, we should get to the hospital. We assumed that would be because we were birthing a lizard. It's because babies can have their first-ever outside-the-body poop – which is called meconium and can be tarry, sticky, black gunk – inside the amniotic fluid. The reason to get to hospital is that you don't want them breathing that in.

"Oliver inhaled some meconium while in the womb and had to spend his first two weeks post-birth in the hospital . . . but we were able to spend endless hours with him, doing the things we would normally do – hold him, cuddle him, change his diaper, give him a bath, feed him, etc. . . . all under the watchful eyes of many nurses and doctors." – Rochelle, writer, mother of one

To deal with the milder pain of early labour, Diana walked around the Beaches Jazz Festival. Heather biked (I know! Biked?! Imagine the circus-like feat of balance that would be!) around her neighbourhood. Naomi played euchre. She forced her buddies to all come to her house and play the damn game with her until she couldn't take the pain any more, and then they were instructed to scram. Which they gladly did. Leslie said that her early labour felt like a corkscrew turning inside her. It made her have to stop whatever she was doing and lie down. What she was doing was walking about in downtown traffic. Fortunately, gigantic, moaning pregnant women always have the right-of-way.

My early labour started at midnight. It felt like hot, squeezing full-body menstrual cramps that came every fifteen minutes and were intense enough to wake me from a sound sleep with a mumbled "Ooohhh." I assumed I was only in pre-labour, and since I'd been told that pre-labour can last many hours, or even days, I didn't wake Janis.

By 3 a.m., my yogic chanting had turned into "Ohhh God, ohhhh boy." Contractions weren't five minutes apart yet, but they were getting close, and were much more intense. I realized that I was officially in early labour as opposed to pre-labour. I nudged my contraction timer. She bolted awake and grabbed her pad, watch, and pen, "Whassup? Y'okay?" she blurted, her hair literally standing on end.

"It's·begun," I said.

We squealed with delight.

After an hour or so, Janis got me into the tub – no small feat when you're 175 pounds and you're having contractions. The water immediately helped the pain. To distract me between contractions, we discussed the goings-on of the *Big Brother* household.

Reality television may be the curse of our generation. It may promote sickening Republican values like ruthless competition, big engagement rings, greed-motivated sadism. It may put many of us television actors and writers on the streets. And yet, its mindless voyeuristic intrigue is a balm for labour pain.

Active Labour

During active labour, the cervix dilates from four to eight centimetres and contractions are typically longer, up to a minute, and come more quickly, three to five minutes apart.

By 5 a.m., my contractions were five minutes apart and more intense. These were the unmistakable signs of active labour. We paged the midwife.

Sara listened on the other end of the phone as I moaned through a contraction. I felt like I was auditioning for aid. Part of me thought I should play it up a bit, but as soon as the contraction hit, I had no choice but to groan through it as honestly as I could. What Sara heard confirmed that I was in active labour, and she arrived by six.

The contractions were pretty hard to handle at this point, but I'd heard many stories of women who'd been labouring away for six hours and thought they were seven centimetres dilated, and turned out to be two, so I had no expectations. Well, God bless the midwife, she checked me and I had dilated four centimetres. By that point, Janis woke up our basement tenant, Dawn. Dawn had just moved in the month before. Lucky her. Janis asked her to go to 7-Eleven and get some Gatorade and make some toast. Sara had suggested I drink as often as possible, and try to eat before I no longer wanted to.

Just as Dawn was bringing the toast upstairs into the land of the primal scream, she heard me barfing. She turned around and crept back downstairs. Too late.

The contractions now started to get very intense. They came in waves. I'd feel the beginning of one, gently starting, teasing nefariously. There would be a peak of pain, and then the contraction would slowly skulk back down. The peaks kept getting higher and the time between them shorter. The pain was more full-body. I lost all sense of modesty as I wandered about naked, dripping, intoning in full voice to the cosmos.

All through labour, Janis instinctively put her hands on my lower back, applying counterpressure that I believed literally saved my sanity. We communicated mostly without words – since mine had become a strange incantation – and she never left my side. She intuitively spoke at the right moments, and was silently soothing at others. Sara said we were one of the best teams she'd ever witnessed. My inner Hebrew-school nerd sat up at that, hoping to get a gold star, or at least a smelly fruit sticker.

After another four hours, we checked again. The contractions at this point were very intense and frequent and I expected to be at seven centimetres. The midwives were always very respectful when they checked my cervix. Never any of this chatting about SARS or the war as they stuck a gloved hand in. No. It was always preceded by "I'm going to check you now, is that okay? You'll feel a touch now, is that okay?" Of course, it's not really okay, is it? Still, it was sweet of them to ask. The next examination showed me to be dilated only five centimetres. I'd dilated one more measly centimetre in four hours. My heart sank.

To get things going, Sara suggested that I do a few contractions on the "birthing ball." They are literally big plastic balls that you can sit on. They make you sit up very straight in your pelvis, and are great for strengthening your core muscles, the ones that get turned into molten taffy during pregnancy. People pay fortunes in Pilates classes to use these devices. I sat on it, the baby's head moved right onto my cervix, more amniotic fluid gushed out and the contractions were much more painful. After enduring one such super-contraction, Sara asked, "Can you do a few more? These are good, strong contractions."

Good, strong contractions? I thought. What is "good" about these? I bartered with her, "All right, Sara, I'll do one more on the damn ball and then two on my side. Then I'll get on all fours for the next one. Okay?!"

One of the pluses about not having an early epidural is that you get to walk, sit, lie down. I can't remember why and when I moved. I was like a wounded animal. My body took over and moved when it needed. No thought. No time. Just a dance of baby's descent.

One of my favourite positions was bending over in our upstairs hallway, resting my elbows and upper body on the banister, pressing my amniotic-fluid-covered butt against the wall, in an effort to brace myself for the next contraction. My body made a giant, pregnant upside-down L shape. After we got home from the hospital, there was a perfect shiny bum imprint in amniotic fluid on this one particular spot on the wall. I left it there for weeks. It was my mark of power, of survival! My Purple Butt. A wholly unsanitary badge of honour.

Leaving Home

I was ten hours into my labour when we determined that despite our many positions, my cervix wasn't dilating beyond five centimetres. However, since the contractions were now coming every two minutes or less, we decided that we'd better get going to the hospital before travel became too dicey.

I came out onto my front lawn. It was around 10 a.m. on August 19th. It was a clear, balmy, gorgeous day. I viewed it through hooded eyes and a slow fog. My peripheral vision had narrowed to a tunnel. I have no memory of what I managed to wear. In my mind, I was buck-naked, with amniotic fluid trailing behind me onto the sidewalk. Part of me wished there was a neighbour or at least a dog walker to witness that it was finally happening!

The route to the hospital was 5.14 kilometres. On a good day, making all the green lights, I can get there in about seven minutes. On this day, we hit every single red light and it felt like it took an hour – although it was probably closer to twenty minutes. I was crouched on my hands and knees in the back seat of Sara's little Peugeot. Janis was kneeling beside me with her hands on my lower back as Sara calmly drove to my pleas of "Please, Janis, please, help me."

Behind us all the way was a red van. I kept wondering what he thought of this sight. I wanted to yell, "I'm in labour! Do something!" I couldn't understand how the traffic lights were just carrying on as if everything was normal. Why wasn't the whole world getting out of our way, elevating us over their heads, and lifting me gently to the delivery room?

Eventually we got to the hospital. As I struggled through a contraction in the doorway, someone brought a wheelchair. My moans ricocheting through the lobby, we easily cleared a path to the elevator. Janis pressed floor seven, Labour and Delivery. I was barely holding on. Then someone else got on. He pressed floor five.

I will never forgive that person. If I could have spoken any words in the English language (as opposed to the middle-earth tongue that was coursing out of me), I would have shouted, "Hey, buddy, take another elevator! They come every thirty seconds, fer fuck's sake!" By now, I was not able to look above the height of my seated eye level. All autonomic functions of my body seemed to be shutting down, conserving energy, focusing. As we neared floor five and stopped, a contraction hit and I started to cry. It was the only time I cried during labour. I don't know why, beyond the deep disappointment that the world wasn't responding to my need as I believed it should. And then an angel spoke up.

In front of me, someone shifted into my sights. He was wearing a white lab coat, white buttoned-down shirt, and yellow tie. "You're almost there," he said. "Two more floors to go. You can make it. You're almost there." He kept repeating those words until the elevator door opened at floor seven and Janis wheeled me out. As the elevator doors closed, he said, "You're doing it. You're there." To whoever you are, thank you.

We breezed through what is normally the triage, where I assume some heretofore unknown nurse would have checked my cervix had I not been with a midwife. We blew into labour room ten, a spacious gymlike room with soft brown cinder-block walls and a bed, cot, baby warmer, and . . . a shower.

By this time my sister was there. Laura was the only other person I wanted in the room with Janis, Sara the midwife, and me. The rest of our family and David were to stay in the waiting room. My plan was that they would get regular reports, but were not to come near the delivery room. I wanted to protect my privacy and did not want to be worrying about other people worrying about me.

During a particularly delightful contraction that seemed to go on for an hour, Sara asked, "Did someone stick a towel under the door?"

"Ohhhh God! Ohhhh man! ohh – what?" I asked.

Unbeknownst to us, someone had wedged a towel under the door in order to keep it propped partially open. Presumably because they were out there and they wanted to hear what was going on. In fact, David was outside the delivery room, excitedly listening at the door and videotaping. My mother was also out in the hall, quietly sending me Reiki. They were clearly on *shpilkehs* and unable to sit still. I have to admit that once I knew someone might be listening (much less videotaping, oy!), I couldn't help but have the tiniest bit of self-consciousness and performance anxiety. I could suddenly hear my own voice and imagine how it sounded to them.

"I outlawed anyone in the delivery room except my midwife, my best friend, and my partner. But my mom got in, told the nurses at the station that she was a nurse herself (which she was), and started to shout at me to breathe. At one point my mom pulled a full-on Shirley-MacLaine-in-*Terms-of-Endearment* fit. She yelled at the nurses that her daughter was: 'In pain! Do something! Give her something!' I had wanted no intervention, and I was doing okay. Managing the pain, going into the tub, using breathing. But my mother's panic made me panic, and I got an epidural." – Farah, mother of one

---

So, a tip, if someone asks you to stay clear of their delivery, don't take it personally. There is so much else you can do for the family once the baby comes! This is an often once-in-a-lifetime event. Respect the mother's wishes.

Back in the delivery room, my contractions were relentless. The tumult of the car ride had kicked them into high gear. We made for the shower. Laura turned the water on, I got on my hands and knees and let the hot stream rush hard onto my lower back. It immediately calmed some of the intensity of the contractions.

Then I made a mistake. Here is the advice I would give to mountain climbers and mothers who are in the showers in hospital labour rooms: Don't look down.

The concrete floor felt and looked a little grungy. I snapped into full princessy consciousness for a brief moment. "Ich," I said, "can someone get me a towel for my hands, this floor is covered in *E. coli*." A second later I forgot what *E. coli*, much less the floor, was.

Shortly after the shower I threw up. It was an iridescent green. In between contractions, I asked Sara why it was green. She answered calmly, with the Zen assurance that we loved, "Because you've been drinking blue Gatorade and yellow Gatorade." I was floored. "She is not only a superwoman," I exclaimed, "but she also knows her colour combinations." Then back to raw, unashamed work.

By noon, a full twelve hours into labour, I was still at five centimetres. This is sensitively referred to as "a failure to progress." I had failed. To progress. With the "getting the baby out" part. Despite all my studying of the phases, this labour would not follow the rules.

Many women get stuck at different points in labour. Especially first-time mothers. Leah was stuck not dilating beyond a few centimetres, and her contractions were continuous. Meaning no break at all in between. After thirty-three hours in labour, her OB came into the room to check her progress. With her gloved hand poking Leah's cervix, the OB proclaimed, "It's a swan's egg in a duck's body. Let's cut her." And did a C-section. The baby was almost nine pounds. I guess this is where the expression "You can't get a swan out of a duck" came from.

Epidural

It was recommended that I have an epidural, and if things didn't progress in another three hours, a picotin drip, to kick it into high gear.

You didn't have to ask me twice. Epidural? YES·PLEASE. What they don't tell you is that it's not like taking an Aspirin.

They have to record twenty consecutive minutes of fetal heart-beat. The heartbeat monitor was possessed, it would cut out inexplicably and we'd have to start over, so that took about two hours.

As we waited for the monitor to record the baby's heartbeat, my sister joined Janis at the low-back pressure application. Unfortunately, she didn't have the perfect touch that Janis had. Even amid the labour pain, I didn't really want to correct my little sister. I didn't want to be bossy. Also, I figured that, Jeez, if I can withstand labour pain, then I can handle some tweaking, can't I? Apparently not. In the midst of an intense contraction, accompanied by moaning and writhing and gripping of hands, I turned to Laura and said, "Could you please not pinch my back fat?"

Then the short, handsome, curly-headed Adonis anaesthetist came in with the needle. The long, very thin needle that goes in your spine. For him to administer it properly, I would have to sit upright, while excruciating contractions racked my body. He said, "Do not move, or this needle could go into the wrong part of your spine and paralyze you for life." You'd think with odds like that, people would not get epidurals. That tells you how much labour hurts.

They asked me to ponder the risks. I actually thought it through: I could still be a mommy in a wheelchair. At least I wouldn't feel this any more. Then I thought that God would punish me for thinking these kinds of thoughts and I would regret this moment of flippant decision-making for the rest of my life. Then another contraction hit and I said, "Gimme gimme gimme!"

At least they *informed* me of the risks. Janis's mother, Doris, was merely told to lie on her side.

"They didn't mention that I should stay still. Luckily, I did. The dose of epidural was so high that my legs became immobile. I remember the nurses hoisting me to a bed, with these two leaden weights that once were my legs, attached to my waist."

In order to remain perfectly still while the needle went into my spine, I had to sit up, with my legs hanging over the side of the bed, and my arms around my partner's neck, resting on her shoulders. She had to wear a mask to prevent infection. As each contraction came, it took all my will not to move or to moan too loudly, so that my back muscles would stay still.

At one point, after the needle was almost out, I realized that Janis was breathing really heavily. It reminded me of Darth Vader. I half expected her to say, "Luke . . . Luke, I am your lesbian mother." What was going on? Then I felt her knees buckle a little. "Stay perfectly still," the anaesthetist murmured, "we're almost done."

I saw beads of sweat on her forehead. Her skin went white. It was then that I realized what a courageous and devoted partner I had. She needed to faint. She was, in fact, in the process of fainting. She *willed* herself to stay conscious, with me.

"Almost done, you can move a little now," said our Adonis.

"Laura, take over," gasped Janis. Laura stepped between my arms and rested them on her own shoulders, as Janis ducked out. Janis hit the floor, got up, and bent into the sink to vomit. Then came back to my side.

We did it.

The epidural worked slowly, and a warm swell of relief started to spread across my body in an uneven ebb. Finally, there was just one tiny nickel-shaped area on the left side of my lower belly that wasn't frozen. It felt like someone was repeatedly stabbing it with a hot knife. "What *is* that?!" I asked Sara, "And how can we make it stop?"

She explained that that was all that was left of the contraction pain. One tiny, localized spot. The intensity of that drop of pain put the whole thing in perspective.

People had warned me that one of the down sides of having an epidural was that you couldn't move. I *was* able to move my legs, and frankly, after fourteen hours of labour and no sleep I was happy to just lie there.

Other Forms of Pain Management

Studies show that the most effective way people can cope with pain is by knowing that it ends. Janis said to me at one point in my last weeks of pregnancy, "Look at it this way, the average woman is in labour for twenty-four hours, so once it starts you'll know that by that point the next day, it'll be over." For some reason that was not at all reassuring.

A number of women I spoke with laboured without epidural, some in tubs at home, some in hospital with labours that moved too fast for anaesthetic to be viable. They all managed and have lovely babies. Most would not have had it any other way. Though, I have to admit, not many of them have had second kids.

Alternate forms of pain management include laughing gas, hypnosis, Demerol, and the TENS machine.

"Do you know what a TENS machine is? In case you don't, I'll tell you, it's these wires and electrodes that you put on your back, or other painful areas, and you control them with a remote. You can increase the intensity of the waves and it's supposed to confuse the brain into thinking you have no pain. A lot of people use them to deal with back pain. Well, I had heard about it in prenatal class, and I borrowed one for my delivery. We also took New Age tapes and pillows from home. Needless to say, once the picotin drip started kicking in at top speed and the contractions were coming fast and furious, I was ripping those electrodes off and screaming for the damn anaesthetist!" – Leslie, mother of four

For the record. I'm glad I felt everything that I felt. But I don't know that I need to feel it again.

The Wait

Sara suggested that we get some sleep and she would check my cervix in three hours. If there was no change, we'd have to induce stronger labour with oxytocin in a picotin drip. Janis lay down beside me, Laura went off to get some sushi for lunch, Sara stayed with us in the room, had a Snickers bar, and did some reports. I remained awake, unable to slip into dreamland.

Laura came back a few minutes later, sushi in hand, to report that my parents and brother and the baby's father wanted to come and see me. I felt bad for them out in the waiting room all this time, so I caved. Ian told us later that the waiting room had been packed with families, and that there was only one pay phone. "That phone alone could finance the entire hospital for a week," he said.

Once everyone came in, they were, naturally, excited and wanted to talk. I was preternaturally happy to oblige. Looking back, I should have just kept that calm little bubble of Sara, Janis, Laura, and me, and maybe drifted off. If I had known what was to come, I would have.

Later, I did try to sleep, and while I was dozing, I felt my mother standing beside my bed. She said that she would like to do some Reiki on me. Would I mind? I didn't have the heart to say, "Actually, I prefer my spiritual healing done by strangers." So she sent her warm energy to me, as she had been doing tirelessly, selflessly for hours in the waiting room.

Sara checked my cervix again after three hours and saw that I was still only dilated to five centimetres. In Ontario, midwives can handle all aspects of birth and newborn care. If there is need for a medical intervention (an epidural, an induction, a C-section), the midwife has to call in the obstetrician on duty to check you. The hospital staff performs the medical intervention, and after the procedure is done, the midwife regains control of her patient. In Quebec, if any intervention is required, the midwife must relinquish control and decision-making. The labouring woman becomes the OB's patient, and the midwife (and all your well-thought-out birth plans) is relegated to the sidelines.

Sara believed that I should have the picotin drip and that we should leave me for a few hours to see if I dilate enough to push the baby out on my own. She could not implement this strategy by herself. She needed a consult. Sara called in the OB on duty to ask what *he* recommended we do. The OB looked at me and said, "Well, I recommend we start the drip, and check her in a few hours. Let's see if she can push this baby out on her own." What a good idea.

They hooked up the drip to an IV. So I had had an epidural, an IV of fluids, picotin, and some antibiotic because I'd developed a fever. Now I just had to wait.

Since I couldn't sleep, we played a game. We started talking about some of the revoltingly onomatopoeic phrases and words that describe birth and pregnancy, like *placenta* and *colostrum*. We decided that they'd be really good band names:

- The Mucus Plugs – a 1980s punk band
- Bloody Show – a British oompah band
- Vernix – a New Wave electronica group
- Meconium – a heavy-metal cover band
- Perineal Massage – a teeny-pop boy band
- The Ring of Fire – a Johnny Cash tribute band
- And my favourite: Failure to Progress – Seattle grunge

We waited, and Sara waited with us. In the end, we had our midwife by our sides for a full twenty and a half hours. From 6 a.m.

Monday until 2:30 a.m. Tuesday. If we had been in hospital, we would have gone through three shifts of OBs, whom we would probably never have met before. Once again, I bless the midwives! They are not touchy-feely granola hippies, they are adrenalin junkies, extreme-sports Olympians!

Even if you are labouring with the pain relief of an epidural, labour is still a momentous experience, and a lot of work. Midwives understand this, but others may not. Family and friends may be tempted to casually drop in or out. Not a great idea.

> "Andy left me at the hospital in labour with Jeremy while he decided to go out for something to eat. He called me from the restaurant where he was enjoying a leisurely lobster dinner. . . . I also remember being in the labour room and having my dad show up late at night to 'keep me company.' I was sitting there listening to him complain about his life and trying to figure out how I could get him to leave." – Michelle, mother of three

> "My husband came in to the delivery room at one point to ask how much longer I would be. Did I have any idea how much they were charging for parking across the street? $4.25 a half-hour! I sent him home." – Lisa, mother of one

Transition
This occurs when you've dilated to eight centimetres and need to get to ten in order to start pushing. Women have told me that these last two centimetres are the most painful part. The time when almost everyone says, "I give up! I can't do this! Get it out another way! I'm backing out!!"

Luckily, I had the epidural at this point, so I coasted through it. Netty felt that she would die during transition. Her whole body was convulsing. Contractions are longer – more than a minute in length – and although for many women there is a break in between, for her they were back to back. Many women throw up in transition, have diarrhea, and are very hot or cold. It can last moments or hours. The only good news is that soon you will be getting to the best part.

STAGE TWO

The Best Part – Pushing the Baby Out

During the pushing stage, which the midwives say can last from ten minutes to three hours, the contractions are forty-five to seventy seconds long and come two to five minutes apart. They are accompanied by an overwhelming urge to bear down.

After a few hours of the picotin drip, I had dilated to ten centimetres and was ready to push. Our second midwife, Joyce, the one who would be responsible for the baby, was paged and arrived in moments.

I was pumped and ready. I told Sara, "I'm going to be really good at this." Years of physical training as an actor had helped me to be able to articulate specific muscles in my body. I also learned how to breathe deeply, which was very helpful throughout.

Although the epidural numbed the pain of the contractions, I could clearly feel the baby's head going down across my tailbone. Then I felt this incredible pressure. I wondered, Could The Bean break my tailbone? Followed by, good God, could this baby come out of my bum?! Other women birth vaginally, but my little baby must have managed to scoot into my intestines and now would like to exit that way! Then that passed and I began to feel the baby's head in my vagina. I had the urge to push.

During pushing, the baby's head rocks toward the front of the vagina and then recedes. You push and it inches down a bit more, and then recedes again. During this time, Joyce asked if I wanted a mirror so I could see the head when it came forward. That presumably helps motivate you to keep pushing so it doesn't recede again. I did take a peek, but then I needed to concentrate on pushing, without being distracted by any other stimulus. Especially if it looked like a hairy grey golf ball.

After much peeking and receding, the head finally sticks in the vaginal opening, which is called crowning. The head stays in place and this is when you need to pant and not push. It is often also called the "ring of fire" – what people refer to when they talk about the impossibly ridiculous pain of birth. What Joan Rivers described as trying to pull your lower lip over your head. In my case, the epidural did not block this pain at all.

I remember thinking, There must be another way. Okay, where's the guy? The guy with thing? The thing that gets this out another way. I mean, you're kidding me, right? Sara kept saying, "Push into the pain, push into the pain." I wanted to yell, "How about I push *you* into the pain!"

If there was any way to back out at this point, I would have taken it. What kept me going was Janis's face, the pure wonder. Every time she got another glimpse of the veiny purply skull, the amazement in her face made me desperately want to get the whole baby out, to share her awe. Despite the pain, that moment was magic, when we realized we were actually there, about to meet our baby!

"I had my baby in water at home. We rented a big tub and I had no pain medication. Just the midwives. I was doing really okay. When the baby was crowning, I was suddenly terribly afraid. I felt that if I did push this baby out, I would explode. I had an image of bits of my body splattering against the wall like a Jackson Pollock painting. Then I just had this thought, I've had a good life. If I'm going to die now, it's okay. And I let go. I released all the fear and tension. Well, that baby flew out." – Chrisanthe, mother of one

Some mothers I spoke to had very long pushing stages – one pushed for six hours and then her baby had to be schlepped out with vacuum suction. He was born with a blood blister the size of an egg where the vacuum had done its work. Doctors will usually not let it go for more than three hours, but the midwives monitor the fetal heart rate, and if everything is fine, they will let you keep trying.

There was a tiny break in the work after my baby crowned. I was relieved that I'd managed to get The Bean to the doorway. Now we had to be careful. Sara put olive oil and hot compresses around my perineum to try to mitigate tearing. I had to push, but stop when told to. Janis later said that she saw the head lodged in there, seemingly with no way out. Then I took a deep breath, and, ignoring the midwives' warnings, gave a big push. Both sides of my labia tore, and the head popped right out.

The notion of tearing sounds gruesome, and although the epidural had worn off so that I could clearly feel the "ring of fire," the stretching of the perineum was so intense that I could not actually sense the tearing. I just felt relief that the watermelon was out of the hole, so to speak.

Janis said it was an unearthly sight. The baby's pale blue head was perched there, outside of my body, moving, turning, while the rest of the baby was hidden inside.

Once the head was out, delivering the rest of the baby was supposed to be easy. We were told that the baby's body flops out, the placenta is pushed out, and you hold your baby, let it nurse, and the next thing you know they're in college.

It didn't quite work out that way. First, before the baby's body could slide out effortlessly and painlessly, there was one thing that still needed to wedge its way out of my hoo-haw. Two things, actually. The baby's shoulders. Nobody told me how much that would hurt! After the head, I relaxed, assuming the real pain was over, and then the football pads came through. Oy.

After that, the baby really did slide right into the midwife's hands. Janis could not believe how long he was. More and more of the baby kept sliding out. Unfurling, like a magician's hanky from his pocket.

"It's the baby!" I said, woozy and triumphant. I could hear the sounds of suctioning. Joyce was getting the amniotic mucus out of its mouth and nose. We waited, terrified, as no other sound came. Finally, thankfully, a cry. A loud, clear cry! Our Bean had arrived.

And then I asked the question that every mom all over the world asks after she's pushed her baby out: "Did I poo?"

The answer, of course, is: "Just a little one." Which, of course, is a lie.

"What is it?" we asked.

"A boy!" said Joyce.

It's not a baby, or a Bean, or an it. It's a boy. A little person! Ours! We wept with joy.

The midwives clamped the umbilical chord and withdrew a small amount of blood, rich in stem cells, which we had decided to save for our baby. In case, God forbid, I hate to even say, but you never know, something should happen, all's well, *k'nein a hora*.

The midwives gave Janis a pair of scissors to cut the chord. It was a thick, hard, bloody mess, but she managed it. The baby was free. And she had freed him. Seconds later, I was holding our child. Our beautiful, pointy-headed, vernix-covered, squishy-nosed, perfect child!

Joyce did a quick examination of the baby called an Apgar test, named after physician Virginia Apgar. She checked heart rate, respiratory effort, muscle tone, reflex irritability (a.k.a. the "don't bug me" response), and colouring. They do it one minute and five minutes after birth and give your baby a score from one to ten. A score of seven to ten is considered normal. Janis and I, even in our exhausted states, couldn't help but think, Score! Go! Get a seven! He scored eight at one minute and nine at five minutes.

Once again, The Bean answered my fears with a clear and present kick.

STAGE THREE
Birthing the Placenta

Laura ran to tell the people in the waiting room the news. However, they couldn't come in until I delivered the placenta and got stitched up. No sweat. I pushed, but the placenta didn't come. I pushed for another ten minutes. Nothing. The midwives gave me an injection of oxytocin to stimulate contractions. Nothing. Sara tugged gently on the umbilical chord. Joyce's face clenched. "You could tear it," she whispered. They stopped and had a hushed conference. Janis looked worried at the sight of so much blood.

The placenta needs to release from the uterus so that it can contract, curl in on itself, and seal itself off in order to stop the bleeding. If the placenta doesn't come out, or come out fully, a woman can hemorrhage or get an infection. Not so many years ago, this was a way women died in childbirth.

The midwives knew it wasn't advisable to wait more than forty-five minutes for the placenta to come out, due to blood loss. So they decided to keep trying until then, after which they would have to call for medical intervention. In that case, the placenta would have to be removed manually, i.e., by hand. I couldn't grasp the concept. Someone would have to put their hand inside my guts and fish something out? It seemed impossibly medieval.

"Well, some guy must come with some thing. It must come out another way," I once again assured myself.

Janis went out to the waiting room to go tell everyone that they couldn't come to see the baby yet. She told them that he was fine, gorgeous, healthy, clearly a genius, but that I was having trouble birthing the placenta, and they'd all have to wait. She didn't tell them I was bleeding, out of it, afraid, and torn open. She didn't want to betray how frightened she was. My mother did understand the gravity, and she instantly ceased her excited planning and classic worrying: "They shouldn't put a birth announcement in the paper in case, God forbid, someone could get their address and do God knows what." Instead, she suddenly got very, very quiet. After all, I'm *her* baby.

David followed Janis from the waiting room and asked that he be allowed to have special time alone with the baby first, before my family. She told him that she had to worry about my needs at the moment and that she'd let him see the baby when everyone was all right. She turned around and walked back to labour room ten, and burst into tears. Joyce put her hand on Janis's shoulder and whispered, "She's going to be fine." Janis later said that she felt like she was cracking apart, which made her worry that she was letting me down, which brought on more crying.

To reassure partners, Janis's tears made me feel cared for, not frightened. Let it out, Pops.

I do understand where David was coming from with his request. I desperately wanted to see and hold my baby too. Unfortunately, I had a job to do. Every few minutes Sara or Joyce would ask me to push. At one point I heard a sound like "Fffwaaaap!" I saw blood splatter across Sara and Joyce's shirts. It looked like someone had soaked a brush in red paint and swung it at them. "Was that the placenta?" I asked hopefully.

"Nope," said Joyce cheerily. She efficiently stripped off her now-blood-stained yellow cardigan and brought over a new blue hospital gown for herself. They kept at it.

Finally, the midwives decided they had to call in the doctors. A few minutes later, six medical staff burst in. Our cozy dark room was flooded with fluorescent lights. Sara and Joyce's quiet, respect-ful whispers were replaced with barked orders and conversation about me but not including me. "Top up the epidural, give her some nitroglycerin."

Janis took our son and instinctively shielded him from it all.

"All right, doctor, put your hand in there. Can you feel it?" instructed the older OB to the young, bespeckled resident.

"Yes."

"Try to get it all out in one go."

"Oops," said the petite intern with her hand in my uterus.

I looked at Janis. My body was convulsing. I was vomiting. My lips were chattering and blue. "Oops?"

Janis was holding the baby, tears streaming down her face. I noticed her tears and mumbled, "Aw, you love your baby?"

"No . . ." She shook her head, "Yes, but no." And she handed him to Laura so that instead of the baby, she could hold my hand.

Later, she joked that it looked like a scene from a bad horror movie. She could see the doctor's hands inside the skin of my abdomen, reaching around and pulling – blech.

In three tries they got the placenta out. They pieced it together to make sure nothing was left inside. My uterus could now start to seal itself off, stopping the bleeding.

Before the birth, I had told the midwives that I wanted to see the placenta. Although I didn't want to take it home, name it, and bury it under a tree, I was curious to get a boo at this remarkable life-sustaining organism. After they removed it, the doctors just dumped it in a metal tray and immediately started stitching me up, chatting all the while.

Sara's face was red, which was the only way I could tell that she was very angry. Always our advocate, she asked the doctors when they'd be done.

"Oh, you don't mind if we just finish stitching her up, do you?"

She obviously did. She wanted to resume my care. As it turned out, I would have suffered much less postnatally if she could have stitched me up herself with the midwife clinic's thinner, more organically comfortable stitches.

Although I was peripherally aware of the politics going on around me, my overwhelming feeling was "Thank God that's over . . . now gimme my boy!"

MEET THE FAMILY

After I was sutured, and two hours after he was born, I finally got to nurse our son. He was so beautiful, so tiny, and he smelled like heaven, where we were sure he had been waiting. He found my nipple and started to nurse with a big wide mouth. It felt like I'd had him forever. Janis gave me Gatorade, and I gave the baby colostrum. It was the perfect eco-circle. (Colostrum is a thick, yellowy liquid full of protein, antibodies, and calories. It is a growth and health elixir that looks and feels a tiny bit like snot. Your baby will live on it for the first few days.)

I wouldn't say that I was instantly in love with my baby, but I did know that I would lay down my life for him. He was so unprotected and such a fierce little soul. Look what he had just gone through to join us out here in the world!

> "I felt that I would die or kill for my son within the first five seconds. For my husband, it took him longer to bond. Twenty minutes." – Rona, mother of one

Joyce had rescued the placenta from the stainless-steel tray and was piecing it together again for me to look at. The tree of life, veined and full of hope. I marvelled for a millisecond, but by that point Laura could not hold the waiting throngs back. Everyone piled in.

The introductions of our son to his world are a blur for me. I know that snapshots were taken, family posed. David, Ian, my parents and sibs got to watch the baby's full physical exam while I was helped to a sitting position and fed warm, sweet tea by Janis and Sara.

Ian later said that the scene reminded him of the movie *Weekend at Bernie's*. To him I looked like a lifeless corpse being hauled into this position for a picture, then flopped into that pose for someone else's camera. "Everyone forgets the mom," Ian sighed, shaking his head.

I remember smiling what I thought was a triumphant, toothy, movie-star smile for the camera while the baby nursed. When I later saw the photo, I was shocked. My face was swollen and ghastly white. My eyes were yellow slits. My celeb-on-the-red-carpet smile was a depleted, one-sided tremble. My expression was one of pure exhaustion. And naked power.

A STUDY IN CONTRASTS

To contrast my experience, I was at the birth of my sister's son through a C-section the following year. She had had numerous ultrasounds that indicated that her baby could be huge – her ultrasound technician estimated twelve pounds. This and the unscientific facts that she was thirteen days late, was five-foot-one and had also become five-foot-one around, and her husband is a giant, made a vaginal birth seem unwise. She had paid through the nose for prenatal care at a birth centre that included midwives (something we got for free in Ontario) and was terribly disappointed that she wouldn't get to continue with their care.

Laura was booked into the hospital for 11 a.m., at which time she was whisked away to be prepped and given an epidural. Her husband, Todd, and I put on sterile hats and gowns and waited to be called into the operating room. We joked that he was going to pass out and I'd have to carry all 270 pounds of him from the O.R. We bashed each other on our fuzzy hair nets with our plastic mittens.

When we were called in, we sobered instantly. He sat by Laura's head, shielded from the view of her mountainous belly by a small operating screen. The room was surprisingly large and was populated with many nurses, anaesthetists, and her surgeon. He was a genial man in his sixties with a soft but frank manner. He told Todd that he could choose not to look at the surgery. Todd held Laura's hand and concentrated on her face. I sat by the screen. I wanted to see the baby arrive.

A small incision was made along Laura's bikini line. Her abdomen was pulled open and amniotic fluid gushed out. A moment later, just like in the pushing phase, the doctor hurriedly got the baby's head out and pulled. It took some strength to get that baby out of the narrow space created by the incision but he finally glided out like a little seal.

He was nine and a half pounds, with a large, perfectly round head.

The doctor lifted Laura's uterus up and sat it on her now empty stomach. He painstakingly stitched up each layer of muscle and tissue. It was an unnerving sight. I couldn't look away. The uterus was a huge, football-shaped organ, taut with muscle. What a marvellous living house. Now here it was, flopped on its side for all to see, being sown and discussed with cavalier. I saluted it once, for its valiant job, and got back to congratulating Laura and meeting her big baby boy.

Laura had only been in the hospital for about an hour and a half; however, she had her complications too. Her baby developed a murmur. There was concern about his breathing and heart rate. He had to be kept in an incubator, with tubes running into his little skull, arms, and legs. It was a traumatic sight. Laura went and nursed him, held him, touched him. Apparently it is common for

C-section babies to exhibit these symptoms, although no one told us that. Three days later, her son was pronounced healthy and sent home with his mom and dad.

At first, Laura's recuperation from her C-section was much faster than mine was after Eli's vaginal birth. Her recovery lasted longer though, while her stomach muscles slowly reached out for each other and knitted themselves back together. She was left with a thick bikini line scar, but as she said, "The last time I wore a bikini I was five." My scars are only available for perusal by Janis and my lucky gyno.

AFTER THE BIRTH – THE FIRST TWENTY-FOUR HOURS
There was one last tussle that Sara had with the doctors. They had had to catheterize me when the epidural was given. After the birth, the doctors wanted to keep the catheter in place, and have me remain in hospital for at least a day. I still had a fever, so they were concerned about infection. Sara thought we should be able to go home as soon as my course of IV antibiotics was finished and I could prove that I could pee on my own. So she asked that the catheter be removed. She made everyone but Janis leave the room. The nurses clucked and shook their heads. "She'll never be able to do it, after what she's been through."

Janis helped me down from the bed into a wheelchair. Sara wheeled me into the bathroom and helped me onto the toilet. She said, "I will stay here with you until you can pee." She turned on warm water. I put my hand under the flow. I waited. Made some jokes about Niagara Falls and the fact that now Sara probably had to pee. We waited. I felt a trickle coming. Panicking, I sent a message to my vaginal muscles to tighten, but there was no response. Those muscles had shut down in protest. Hot and burning, the pee finally came. I did it. We were so proud!

I did tell Sara that I intended not to poo again. I swore that nothing else would be pushed out of me again, ever. She advised me that sometimes the secret is not in the pushing, but in the relaxing. Indeed.

We changed our son into the outfit that we had chosen. A cap was put on his pointy little head, and he was swaddled tightly in a receiving blanket by the instructive Joyce. Our families left, and Janis and I, the new moms, were taken to a hospital room up in the maternity ward. It was 2:30 a.m. and we were informed that despite my formidable feat of *pishing* on my own, we had to wait until the following afternoon for my IV of antibiotics to be done in order to leave. Sara was disappointed, but in hindsight, it was the best thing that could have happened to us. A cot was wheeled in for Janis. I was helped into bed and untangled from my IV chords. The attending nurse was surprised that I didn't have a catheter. "You can pee?!"

"Yeah, baby," I swaggered, my IV pole clinking against the bed rails.

Our son was put into a bassinet in the room with us. The new family slept. Together at last.

Our baby slumbered peacefully for hours, exhausted from his traumatic entry into the big world from his warm water cave. We tried to sleep. I admit that I was mostly unsuccessful. I kept waking up and looking at Janis's exhausted blissful smile, and listening for the sweet, rapid, irregular cooing of our little one. It didn't help that they woke me up to nurse him every two hours, and to check on my IV in the hour in between.

By 6 a.m. we decided to give up and just stay awake. A new shift of nurses came by, exclaimed, "You can pee?" and then helped us breastfeed. We couldn't quite figure out how to make him latch. Our nurse sat me up straight, took the baby's lower jaw, opened it wide, and smooshed his face forcefully onto my breast. She looked at him. Nope. Not a good latch. She stuck her baby finger into his mouth, unlatched him, and smooshed him hard onto my breast again. She showed us the "football" hold. You rest the baby on your forearm like a football, with his head under your breast and push him up and on. We needed both of us to make this happen.

"Do you think he's sucking? Can you feel his tongue?" Janis asked.

"I have no idea." I confessed, "Can you tell if he's swallowing? Are his ears moving?"

"Aha! Yes, he must be getting some."

What a team! We became a well-oiled pit crew. "You hold his head, I'll open his mouth. Okay, push him on! Get him on! Gooooo, on!"

We spent the morning lying together in bed, with the baby on our chests, letting him sleep, dropping off ourselves, getting help with breastfeeding, getting fed ourselves. The nurses would not let visitors in for a bit, and then promised that they'd limit the number and time of the visits for us. That morning, it was just the three of us. It was a perfect little envelope of calm. A cherished time.

Janis discovered that there was a breastfeeding seminar with a lactation consultant later that morning. We decided to go. I hadn't got out of bed on my own yet. I felt pretty beat up, but I also felt full of adrenalin. I stood up. No problem! I made jokes about my stitches, my big boobs, my squishy baby-free stomach, I felt like *me*!

I shuffled into the hallway. Janis said that she'd join me in a minute with the baby, since I had to push my IV pole. I set off confidently down the hall. Sure, the stitches hurt, my legs were weak, but I was moving.

By the time I got twenty feet, I had begun to shake uncontrollably. My knees were wobbling. My mouth was dry. My head was swimming. My body was cold and desperately trying to sink to the floor. The forty more feet down the hallway seemed like a mile. I could barely utter "Help." Janis came and took my arm. We walked at an appallingly slow pace to the breastfeeding seminar. I sank into the plush peach couch, exhausted, sweating, stunned. I expected sore muscles, pain from stitches. I'd heard the joking, "You'll need to sit on an ice doughnut." I figured I'd bounce back as I had always done. I had no idea how intense the physical recovery would be.

During the breastfeeding class, we realized that we were the only ones there whose baby had been born within twenty-four hours. Everyone else had been there a few days. They looked at us like we were nuts for even moving. "You can *pee*?!" They gawked.

Then we noticed a woman with tiny twins. One was on each breast. Her partner held one of the baby's heads in place. Janis and I looked at each other, silently grateful to only have to struggle with one. We bow to all you mothers of multiple births.

Janis and I watched the instructor (who, when she saw that my other half was a woman, smoothly switched from saying "your husband" to "your partner") manipulate a lifelike doll into a number of positions. She explained how the sucking worked, that they don't actually *suck*, their tongues *lick* forcefully, which stimulates the milk ducks to let down the milk. Babies won't suffocate under your breasts, their noses are shaped specifically to allow them to take in air under there. They have to get part of your breast tissue in their mouths, not just the nipple, which is why it's called *breast*feeding. Armed with all this information, and the visual of the instructor's baby dummy, we hurried at a snail's pace back to our room.

Forty-five minutes later, the well-wishers started coming. Those who were already parents, like Ruth, knew enough to bring chocolate croissants, weep subtly with joy, and leave after twenty minutes.

David came and stayed much of the day. He was plotzing with love and pride. He brought his cameras and his closest friend, Cyd, and her mother. They brought pastries and toys and *mazel tovs*. They couldn't help but remark how much the baby looked like David. The baby really did have his father's exact hairline (slightly receding – in a rakish way) and shape of face. I have to admit that

I was disappointed. David is handsome, so it wasn't that. I just worked so hard, and wanted some sort of instant kudos. My family came with food and love, and declared that the baby looked exactly like . . . my father.

It's hard to know whose place it is to come to see the baby in the hospital the next day, or even in the first week. If you need to question whether you are close enough to be one of those people — <u>you are not</u>. Stay away, you won't be missed, make a glamorous appearance with pizza and a cleaning crew in the next few weeks. You will be a saviour.

Sara came by (only fourteen hours since we'd last seen her) and weighed the baby in a little sling. He hadn't yet dropped from his birth weight. Many babies do lose a few ounces in the first days due to the sudden disappearance of the constant nutrients (womb service) from your umbilical chord. Sara gave us some more tips about breastfeeding — watching my attempts first before stepping in and basically getting us to do it again, but right. She showed us how to swaddle him in a receiving blanket, wrapping our Bean up like a burrito, and helped us give him a quick wash. While we longed to get home and be alone, we were united in our desire to have Sara move in with us for the next fifteen years.

Sara also helped us to figure out how to get our tiny baby into his big car seat, and wished us well. We cried as we waved goodbye to her, but knew that thanks to the civilized Ontario medical system, we would be visited by her again the next day at our house. Now home to three not two.

Despite the fact that our baby weighed only seven pounds and occupied twenty inches of space, he was about to take over.

• • •

As Ruth insists, it doesn't matter how you get the baby out, just that you do. Drugs, drug-free, hypnosis, C-section, tearing, episiotomy, suction, forceps, a big stork, or finding it in a cabbage patch — it's all valid and worth trying. You can cope and you will cope.

• • •

7

The First Few Days

What Hit Me?

*We spent the first days staring into our son's blue eyes, while
he scanned our hairlines and talked to spirits in the sunbeams.*

When we arrived home from the hospital, we were greeted
by a four-foot stork on our front lawn. Its cartoon
thought-bubble proudly exclaimed, "It's a Boy!" Taped
to our front door was a cheery "Welcome Home, Bean!" sign. A
huge bouquet of multicoloured helium balloons waved enthusias-
tically from our porch.

Although I have no memory of this, I am told that when I saw
all these celebratory messages, I burst into hysterical sobs, repeating, "It's a boy. It's a boy. It's a boy" while crying, laughing;
delighted and touched.

Our uber-tenant, Dawn, the witness to this moment, admits
now to being a little concerned for my mental stability. I was
simply amazed that people could be so thoughtful, and that I had
to go through so much pain when a stork could have delivered
him all along!

When we got inside, we immediately realized that something was missing. There was no evidence of the mess of labour. Some brave souls had cleaned the vomit, blood, and amniotic fluid from the floor, changed the sheets and made the bed. The fridge and freezer had been cleaned out and stocked. Angels had been at work.

For the next few months, the angels kept us going. Our wonderful community, friends, and especially our family would pop by with homemade cookies, frozen burritos, Chinese food, flowers. Teresa made veggie curry. Shoshana made muesli that we ate every morning. Sonja and Deb brought fresh blackberries from their garden. These weren't friends that we saw every week, but generous and excited people who welcomed the baby and smoothed the first few months in ways that they can never know.

SPIRITS IN THE SUNBEAMS AND OTHER SURPRISES

The only thing more beautiful than people's kindness was the baby himself, *k'nein a hora*. We were knocked out by the sweetness of his cooing, his scent, his attempts to communicate. He seemed so peaceful, so wise. Then, in the evening of the first day, our placid angel had a sudden, violent session of kicking and bucking, slapping, and yowling. Uh oh. We were at a loss. Janis lay both her arms on either side of his body, and put her face right next to his. "Shhh shh, my baby," she whispered. He calmed instantly, and let one rip.

The newborn's porous digestive systems is what will make the first three months an expedition into the world of gas liberation. The midwives recommended that when our baby displayed signs of being gassy, instead of whacking his back to burp him, we gently press upward along his spine, kneading the gas up as opposed to shaking it up. Another nifty trick was bringing their knees up to their chest and rolling the legs in a little circle. It just looks like it would make them feel better. I would pay a lot for someone to do this to me. The midwives also suggested that we lay the newborn, tummy down, on our knees, so that gas could pass out through either end. These are now methods that I employ for myself and they work spectacularly well. Maybe that's why one of my son's first sentences was "Mama . . . fart."

Our fellow laughed in his sleep on his third day on earth. We were floored. What on earth could be funny already? The wacky birth canal? That hilarious receiving blanket? Or maybe those goofy plants that winked at him in the breeze.

Newborns can only see black and white, so anything with major contrasts excites them and draws them in. Once we got wise to this, we wore checkerboard everything and played with shadows. I'm sure there are moms out there who do the full-on Goth look. I understand. After working so hard to bring him into the world you want to make sure that he's more interested in you than the damn mobile.

Besides staring at him adoringly while he was asleep or awake, our major preoccupations in the first week were breastfeeding and adjusting to sleeplessness. The first night home alone with the baby, he woke up every two hours, and he stayed awake from 1:30 to 3:30 a.m. Welcome, Bean. Now let me explain a concept that we here on earth call *night*.

AND YOUR NAME IS?

Before we could turn him into a diurnal being, we had to know what to call him. We were given some forms to fill out when we left the hospital, including one for his birth certificate and one for the Child Tax Credit (a monthly government stipend, presumably a reward for not going insane and running out on your kid). For both, we needed to put down our child's name. Janis and I had worked out middle, last, and Hebrew names, a tall order given our unique familial situation. But we couldn't decide on the first. We were torn between two. The second name choice, Benjamin, had arrived late on the scene, but was making headway. We left the hospital with him unnamed and gave ourselves a deadline of two days.

On the second day after the birth I just knew. I looked at Janis square in the eyes and said, "He's not Benjamin."

"Okay, sweetie," she said, already by rote.

"He's Eli." I asserted, tears welling. "That's who he is."

"Okay, sweetie," Janis whispered to us both. "Welcome, Eli."

We kept Benjamin as a middle name. (Since then, I've noticed that Benjamin is the bridesmaid of names – always the middle never the first.) Benjamin in Hebrew translates as "son of the right side." We thought it was appropriate. Eli used to lie facing the right in utero, he was born with his head turned to the right, and he tore the f$#@ out of the right side of my labia.

In Hebrew, Eli means ascension, enlightenment in a spiritual way. It also means "my God." Before we had the baby, we thought that was a little religiously bald, a titch spot-on. After going through the miracle of childbirth and nursing, it seemed about right.

DID ANYONE GET THE LICENCE OF THAT TRUCK?

I was blindsided by the effects of childbirth. I had no idea that I would feel like I had just been hit by a car. This sentiment was echoed by almost every woman I spoke with. Many were furious that no one told them how incredibly debilitating birth can be.

It was partially my fault. The first day we were home, we had many visitors. We were so high on new love that we let everyone come and stay as long as they liked. Although it was a trial to go up and down the stairs, and Janis encouraged people to come up to me, I went down a few times to join in living-room conversation. I was trying to be a hip mama. Sittin' there, chilled out, kicking back with my babe. In my bathrobe. Perched on an ice pack. With my stomach like a sack of jam. And my stitched-together Frankenstein Vajuj.

The following morning I could barely move. My stomach muscles were unable to collect themselves well enough to get me to a sitting position without help. My legs were wobbly, head achy, and mind numb. However, I did enjoy stretching out on my stomach again. After nine months, it was delightful to loll about like a seal without anything between my tummy and the sheets. Except those red-hot, swollen tah-tahs . . .

Here's another little secret. Because of stitches, wiping with toilet paper can be painful, unproductive, and unhygienic. So, I was given a peri-bottle. *Peri* is for *perineum*. A Peri-bottle is a water bottle that has a spout with lots of holes, so it can spray in a wider area. Basically, it's a sprinkler for your hoo-haw. Fill it with warm water, and let me tell you, it feels *great*. Many women confided to me that they hung on to that thing long after the stitches were out. It just felt so damn good.

If you have a tear or an episiotomy, your stitches will be pretty uncomfortable. The huge pad you wear for bleeding will make you walk like you just got off a horse. I didn't realize that I would need the mega-sized pad because I would continue to bleed *heavily* for six weeks.

In many cultures women "lay in" for forty days. They are cared for, fed, and given useful instruction by elder women. They get relief in dealing with their newborns so that they too can heal. In our culture, many spouses go back to work after two weeks, leaving an exhausted, traumatized, and depleted mom to care for her baby alone, pushing her dangerously close to postnatal depression.

BABY BLUES

Almost every woman I've spoken with had a bout of what is cutesily referred to as "baby blues." My experience with postnatal depression was shocking, but relatively minor. It appeared sporadically in the first few days and it involved sprawling naked on the bed echoing tonelessly, "I feel nothing." I wasn't able to display an ounce of joy. Yet, hours later, my happy-cup overflowed when I held my son and he looked into my eyes with been-here-before wisdom.

"I put on eighty pounds during my pregnancy. It was mostly water, and I lost almost all of it within the first two months. I was trying to get back to work as well as care for my newborn. This shock to my system sent me into postnatal depression. As a result, I had to take off weeks of work, and found it difficult to bond with my newborn." – Susan, mother of one

Many of the women I spoke with seemed ashamed of the blues. They had an urge to dismiss the effect of this natural phenomenon. An enormous drop in estrogen levels, combined with sleep deprivation, boredom, and stress have got to have some emotional effect, don't they? Why do we feel ashamed?

It doesn't help that unless you can say instantly, "I *looove* my baby. I am filled to the brim with giddiness. It was worth all the pain," you are considered a beast. It is time to let go of the Stepford-mom ideal.

Speaking of idealized images, here is a list of . . .

Ten Odd and Unusual Things About Newborns that Might Give You the Skeevies

1) They don't blink.

Don't have a staring contest with one. You will lose. Your eyes will water, and you will become terrified that your baby's eyes must be dry as a bone and will remain permanently stuck open. They also cry without tears for the first little while. They're not faking it, they just don't have working tear ducts yet. Rest assured, the first real tear that rolls down that sweet, chubby cheek will *kill* you.

2) They poop while they eat.

Somehow, this makes sense to them.

3) They have wobbly dead-turkey necks.

Their neck muscles haven't developed yet, so all the tendons and ligaments are loose enough to allow them to flop their left ears over to their right shoulders. Skeevie!

4) They fling their arms out like little freaked-out bats.

The Moro or Startle Reflex is an adaptive hangover from Cro-Magnon times. If anything sudden happens, a breeze, a light, an errant thought, they are likely to throw their little arms out to the sides and jerk them like they were about to take flight and then thought better of it. I call it the "bat wing" reflex, but a more charitable fellow, Jeff, calls it "Jazz Hands."

5) They curl their feet and hands if you tickle them.

This is also an adorable reflex because if you give a newborn your finger, they will hold it tightly in theirs. The skeevie element of this is that the fingers and toes clench because they are trying to hold on to the fur on their mamas' backs. So, back in Neanderthal days, when you and I were women-who-ran-with-the-wolves, our babies could go for a ride. No slings, Bjorns, or Trekkers, just luscious back hair.

6) They bob their heads like little chickens pecking for food.

This "rooting reflex" helps you know when they are hungry. But you, most likely, are not a bag of grain.

7) They move like mechanical movie babies.

You know those really fake-looking robot babies that they use in films to represent newborns? The ones with the arrhythmic jerky motions? That is what babies actually look like in the first few days. Even yours, who is so cute and precocious and already smiling and saying "Doctoral Thesis."

8) They come out with long, yellow, curling-over-the-edges fingernails.

And they're sharp. Those talons will carve into you and themselves, so you must cut them. That first nail-cut was almost as traumatic as the first bath or the first inoculation. Some people bite their baby's nails off, but I found that even more daunting. I already felt a bit like a cow, I couldn't bear chewing on my baby as well.

9) They have a soft spot on the top of their skull.

They may also have jaundice, cradle cap, and baby acne on their heads and faces. All are normal and will pass. All are also a tiny bit skeevie.

10) They make loud, unearthly piggy noises.

A neighbour e-mailed me in shock soon after her baby came:

"Did Eli ever make extremely odd, loud demonic noises – particularly at night? Oliver makes these staccato, throat-clearing sounds that make him sound like he's possessed. We've checked for horns and don't see any, but those sounds are enough to drive one insane!" – Rochelle

THE FAMILY BED

We had wanted to have the baby in bed with us. Actually, Janis did. I was worried I would squish him in my sleep. After being assured by numerous friends and advocates of "the family bed," we opted to try it for the unromantic reason that it seemed like the easiest thing to do. (Also, then I could more efficiently check every twenty seconds to make sure that he was still breathing.)

The first night that we got home from the hospital, we put him to sleep by my side of the bed in a beautiful rocking bassinet that Richard gave us. Then we got into our bed, intending to pull him in between us when he fell asleep. The pillows were all removed, the duvet was pulled down. There was nothing that could strangle or smother him. We were ready. Unfortunately, just as we got relaxed, Eli started his engines. Sara described our son's newborn sleeping sounds as a cross between an elephant at full-mating trumpet and a car screeching around a corner in an underground parking garage. We couldn't believe it. He was seven pounds! Where was this sound coming from?

"I know it's supposed to be a blissful image – the mom and babe sleeping together, but it's really hard to relax when you're lying next to snorty snorty pig boy." – Lori, mother of one

As most newborns do, he was waking every hour and a half to two and a half hours to nurse. In the little pocket of time that he actually slept, I couldn't sleep because of how loud he was.

After three weeks, we couldn't take it any more. I wasn't getting any sleep at all. So Janis, ever the intrepid one, decided that he had to sleep in the crib in his own room. That meant we lost the convenience of just scooping him up and nursing him in bed. I also couldn't peek and poke at him as easily. Instead, I had to get up, shuffle to the next room, pick him up, sit in a rocking chair and nurse him. And feel his chest to make sure he was breathing. And kiss his hands and feet and belly and little face. This often made it much harder to get back to sleep, but it was worth it.

Top Three Odd and Unusual Things About Newborns that Will Give You the Joyful Weepies

1) The way their heads smell.
2) Their seriously unique personalities (that appear from moment one).
3) They make you live in the present for possibly the first time in your adult life.

BATH TIME

You may well wonder, How dirty can a newborn get? All she does all day is nurse, stare, and burble. Yes, she spits up all over herself.

And, true, trying to get diarrhea off of a baby boy's scrotum is like trying to get butter off of an English muffin.

For sure you don't have to wash his hair. He's not putting product in it. Okay, maybe there's still bits of meconium there from the birth, but that's natural, right? I bet people pay money to coat their babies in that stuff. I support you, sister, in your desire to let nature's healing oils remove crap from your baby's hair; and let the wonder of cellular recycling slowly slough dead skin cells off of your grungy little angel over a period of, say, months.

If you do decide to take the plunge, you'll probably start with one of those cute shallow plastic tubs. Some have cup holders, for your coffee maybe.

Now, the big question: How hot should the water be? I remember asking Sara and she shrugged and said, "Warm, but not what you'd find hot. Probably warmer than you'd think."

How does that help me? I want numbers, I want specific dial settings. We settled on a temperature that was slightly warmer than the neutral feeling you get when you drip warm water on the inside of your wrist.

I was very nervous the first time. One slip and he could breathe in water and get pleurisy or pneumonia and be in an iron lung! Can't babies drown in an inch of water? Even if he has two moms with four hands gripping him? These arguments failed to convince Janis to leave him dirty until he was old enough to sing in the shower. Our midwife assured us that babies don't need to be scrubbed with soap in the first little while. Just a dunk in some water with a little shpritz of baby wash in it was enough.

So, we got everything ready. We undressed him. Brought him naked to the tub. We paused and just looked at him. I hadn't sat and simply looked at my naked child yet. I held him and breathed the scent of him. He gazed up at me (my hairline), then at Janis (her eyebrows). Then he peed on us.

Slowly, slowly, holding his soft, pointy head, we submerged him bit by bit in the water. First legs, then his back, then his arms — being very careful not to let the umbilical stump get wet.

Oh, the caution one takes with the umbilical stump. It's like it's the Hope Diamond instead of a black and yellow putrefying flap of dead skin. We read many different books, with passionately argued philosophies about the stump, to clean or not to clean, using alcohol or none. Some argued that the alcohol was of course necessary to disinfect and speed the drying — dear God, would you let a child's open wound just turn to a pustule?! Other books said that the alcohol would damage the baby's skin and was another example of the medical system's desire to pathologize and control motherhood.

In the end, we went with our midwife's suggestion — just leave it, it'll dry out and drop off on its own — because it was lower maintenance. My sister cleaned her baby's umbilical stump with alcohol every day using a Q-tip. Both my sister's and my son's stumps dropped off at the appropriate time with no fuss. Janis and I barely noticed it, just found it one day on the floor. A blackened nub of skin. Delightful! We celebrated. We wanted to make a party for it. I ended up keeping it wrapped in a drawer for months. One day I found it and freaked out because I thought it was a bug.

Back to the bath. All went well with Eli's first dunk. He kicked a bit. He peed again. We decided not to wash his hair. We took him out and he was fine.

It was not long until I had another test of my comfort zone. Janis decided that she wanted to take him into our big tub with her. I looked at her like she had just suggested we let Eli back the car out of the driveway. She thought it would be a beautiful, bonding experience. My mind raced to all the things that could go wrong, including possible hygiene issues. "Just how clean are *you*?" I squinted at Janis.

After I gave her the Silkwood scrub-down and scoured our tub with natural antibacterial cleansers, we filled the bath with warmish water. Janis got in. I held the baby. I got peed on (by the baby). I gently handed him to her. She cradled him in both her hands and let him lie on his back on her chest. His limbs relaxed. He looked at the dark blue geometric tiles on the white walls. He was fascinated. He kicked his legs happily. There was no mistaking it. He loved it.

BREASTFEEDING

If you've read anything about breastfeeding you will have gleaned that it is *not* natural. It's a sensually lovely and biologically miraculous thing, but it ain't like learning to wink. This is also the time of the largest hormone influx in your entire pregnancy and childbirth. So, besides the stress of trying to keep something that can't talk to you alive, you might be chemically psycho.

At first you need all your powers of concentration, a darkened room, and a team of lactation consultants, nurses, midwives, and partners standing by. It's hard to imagine that in a few months you'll be talking on the phone, typing, eating, and reading a magazine with him on one boob.

For the first few days, I needed help holding his wobbly head, while I gripped my breast and rubbed my nipple over his lips again and again, waiting for him to open up like a baby bird. When he did, we'd jam him on. You have to try to get their lips to be open and pressed up on your breasts, as opposed to sucked into their own mouths. If you can do all that right away, you are freakishly gifted. You should give the rest of us your number. So we can crank-call you.

In the first few days, all the baby is getting is the yellow, slimy, immune-boosting colostrum. By day three or four, you will start to produce breast milk.

When your milk "comes in," you might become what is accurately called "engorged." Your breasts will pop out like animated porn. You thought they were big before – just wait. They might become hot, hard, lumpy, and very sore due to the sudden influx of milk in your milk ducts. You may be lucky and not become engorged at all because you have a body that times things out perfectly. Don't spread this around if you want to remain popular.

The midwives recommend an ancient method of dealing with the swollen, heat-seeking mammaries. Put cold cabbage leaves in your bra. They will slowly suck the heat from your breasts and cool everything down. Although when I first heard this suggestion I rolled my eyes at Sara, "You are such an earth-mama. Why don't I just dip my breasts in mud and chant to the moon?" The *second* I became engorged I found myself moulding two large cold cabbage leaves inside my leopard-patterned nursing bra. It worked! Even though I looked like a vegetarian's nightmare and smelled like borscht.

From a woman who never wore a bra, sometimes not even to workout, I suddenly had to wear one to bed. Otherwise, I risked knocking myself unconscious as I shifted in my sleep, or drowning us all in life-giving, buttery, leaking mama-milk.

Visitor Fatigue

One day in the first week, I was sitting on an uncomfortable, posture-perfect hard-backed chair, Eli's head in my right hand, as I held his body like a football and tried to get him to open his kitten maw wider so he could get a mouthful of my right breast. He was crying and not sucking, and I was fretting.

My nipples were already raw from the times that he latched onto them only, and not the actual breast tissue. My milk had just come in and my breasts were very hot and uncomfortable. I was wearing a robe that wouldn't close properly over my belly. (Janis and I were

in PJs and robes for the first month or so – alternating with each
other for a change of fashion.) My hair had yet to be washed since
the big delivery day, and I could feel blood leaking over the sides of
my mega-pad.

Although I thought my son was latched on, I was uncertain if
he was sucking. I couldn't hear the little clicking sounds that indicate swallowing that Sara had suggested we listen for. David was
kneeling by my breast, singing to Eli in Yiddish. My sister was on
the other side of me, watching intently, and occasionally making a
suggestion directly out of a "breastfeeding is natural" pamphlet
that she was holding. Some friend of mine, a Monday Morning
Quarterback (whose face I have conveniently erased from my
memory), was kneeling below me, tickling the baby's jaw, ears, and
feet in an attempt to force a sucking reflex.

In my mind's eye, there were about a dozen other people there
too, their own mouths latching and relatching like fish as they
watched me try desperately to make a good connection with my
newborn. They were shouting out comments, "Take some of his
clothes off. Stick your finger in his mouth first. I don't think he's
sucking. . . ." Through a haze, I looked at my bed and to my
horror, sitting there, in matching pant suits, was a whole panel of
older women judges holding up scorecards. I think the Russian
judge gave me a two-point-four for technique and a minus six
for style.

Finally I managed to get the baby to suck. Janis came in and saw
the tinge of madness in my eye and shooed the phantoms and
family away. Eli ate, farted, and went to sleep. I collapsed on our
bed in a fetal position and wept, "I need to be alone when I nurse!
I don't know what I'm doing!"

I didn't have to say any more, Janis became a bulldog there and
then. Everyone had to leave while I nursed. No exceptions. Even
if I wanted company. She began to implement a half-hour rule,
which ended up being an hour rule, and to demand that whoever

visits also cleans our bathroom. I thought that was pushing it – but it worked.

Complications

In the first week, quite a number of women I spoke with had dangerous complications with breastfeeding. Some babies latched but didn't suck, or couldn't latch properly at all. Although he seemed to be eating, Netty's son, Parker, kept inexplicably losing weight. It was terribly alarming. Her doctor advised her to use formula. The midwives advised her to keep at it. Lactation consultants advised supplementing with a tube of breast milk. Netty felt like a victim in a turf war. She was exhausted, terrified for her child's life, and needed clear direction about what to do. After feeding Parker with a spoon for the first few weeks, he figured it out and now nurses and eats voraciously.

Jenny and Victoria had a litany of similar struggles: cracked and bleeding nipples, mastitis (a painful fever-causing infection of the milk ducts), baby refusing to latch and becoming dehydrated. They both eventually turned to bottle-feeding and their sons are healthy and thriving. Plus, the moms had the bonus of not being tied to their child twenty-four hours a day.

Ultimately, how you get food in your baby matters little, so long as they get nourishment.

I was lucky. I had a blocked duct that needed to be treated with warm compresses and pressure, but Eli fed like a champ. He lost a few ounces in the first day, and then gained a pound a week for the next six weeks. A Midwife Collective record.

My friends and I had many resources to help us figure this breastfeeding conundrum out. In my mother's day, there were no such luxuries.

"I was given the feeding ritual by the hospital nurses and Dr. Spock. The baby was to be fed every four hours, and be 'taken off the breast' after ten minutes and burped. To stretch out the time between feedings he was to be given water and walked, until the time was right for the next feeding. If he was asleep, he was to be woken up and fed. We couldn't nurse on demand and rooming-in was still a dream. But there were times when the baby needed to nurse more often, and water did not satisfy him, so he was crying and desperate. And sometimes he needed to nurse longer, falling asleep on the breast. When I broke the rules it was a guilty thing. But I did it anyway." – Lily

One final word about breast milk: it's tasty! Before your flow becomes regulated, it can spray all over you and your baby in an excess of production. You might accidentally get a shpritz of the sweet, creamy stuff on your arm. Take a lick. I know you want to.

SLEEP
The other huge challenge with the newborn is sleep. You will soon understand why sleep deprivation is used as a form of torture. After the first few days you will be willing to sign any confession handed to you in any language.

Night means nothing to a newborn. Prenatally, babies sleep in small doses all day and night suspended in your dark, warm womb. Once they're out in the world, they need time to understand that at night, when they wake up to feed, they should be civilized and go right back to sleep. Instead, sometimes they stay up for hours: crying, staring, burping, and needing your help to return them to dreamland.

Friends advised us to think of our sleep time in a twenty-four-hour clock. Go to bed at 8 p.m. and don't attempt to get out until after 11 a.m. Sleep when the baby sleeps, if you can. Doze off when you can't. Then you might get an interrupted eight hours.

"In the beginning, I'd cope by dropping off to sleep any-where by 8:30 p.m. One night, I was woken up from a deep sleep by a phone ringing. 'Who would dare?! It's the middle of the night!' I said. I nudged my husband out of bed to pick up the phone. It was my grandmother. It was 9:30 p.m."
– Lara, mother of one

Life as you know it, Party Gal, is over for a bit. Don't worry, you won't miss it. Your baby is doing all the late-night carousing for you.

Often in the first week, Eli would wake up in the night, nurse, and look around for where the action was. We had to discover what lulled him back to sleep. Janis was walking him back and forth in the hallway one night when she decided to go downstairs to get something. By the time she got back upstairs, he was asleep. Aha! Stairs! So in the night we'd trade off. Janis would do the stairs five times. If Eli wasn't asleep, I'd do another one or two sets, then she'd keep going. Our record was twelve.

Sometimes you just need someone else to take over. One night, at 4 a.m., Janis came into our son's room to find me holding him as he sobbed inconsolably. I was bouncing up and down with a wild look in my eyes and plaintively asking Eli and the universe, "What?! What?! What?! What?! What?!"

Janis carefully pried the baby from my arms, and angled me back to the bedroom. I what-ed myself down the hallway, into bed, and back to sleep.

My sister had an automatic swing. It saved her sanity. She'd pop a crying Jordan in it and, within minutes, he'd be back to sleep. She could leave him there for an hour. Diana, mother to James, lovingly referred to their swing as the "neglect-o-matic."

Necessity is the mother-bear of invention and you will discover your own sleep-inducing tricks. A sampling of tips for when the boob isn't enough include: rocking, bouncing, singing, a noise-machine that makes different womblike shushing sounds, pacifier, running a vacuum cleaner, laying them on a working dishwasher or washing machine, degassing them, calming music (Janis chose something randomly in the first week that we ended up getting stuck with to this day. It's Enya. And it works), putting them in a sling and walking around with them, endlessly, taking them for a drive in the car (good luck transferring them from the car to the house, though), gripe water (a British remedy for colic and other digestive upsets. Aara, from the midwife prenatal group, swore by it. Especially the kind that has a little alcohol in it. When she was once offered one without any alcohol, she said, "Are you, crazy? We _need_ that drop of booze in there!").

NUMBER TWO

Janis and I were advised that since by necessity I had to do all the night feedings, Janis should be responsible for any midnight poo-ey diaper changes. This idea ended up working well for Janis since Eli didn't poo but once a week for months.

We were initially alarmed by this anal retention. (Not to mention the fact that breastfed baby poop smelled swampy sweet, like microwave popcorn.) The books told us that we had to make sure that he peed once on the first day, twice on the second day, and so on, to make sure he was not dehydrating. We assumed the same for poops. When he didn't poop in twenty-four hours, we paged the midwife. She was in the middle of a birth. She left the labouring mother to answer our call.

"Hi, Joyce, I don't know if this is a 'pageable moment' or not, but Eli has not pooped in twenty-four hours!"

"He doesn't have to. If he doesn't poop for five days, then we'll talk." Joyce was reassuring but wanted to get off the phone.

"And then what?" I pushed on, suddenly unconcerned about the needs of a labouring mother who was not me.

"Then we'll wait another five days."

"But hang on, hang on, why isn't he pooping? Where is the milk going?"

"He's digesting it."

With that, she got back to the delivery room. Breast milk is so efficiently pure and usable to the new body that there may be little or no waste.

Your child's poo: the size, colour, frequency, and decibel level can be preoccupying and, occasionally, appalling. Thank God Ruth was with me a few days later when Eli had his first gigantic poop. I was nursing him and he made a sound like "ffrrraaaapffffpowpow!"

"Good boy," Ruth said calmly.

She responded to my bug-eyed look of revulsion by explaining, "They like to poo while they nurse. They're relaxed." I started to get up to change him and Ruth raised one skinny string-bean arm and said sagely, "Wait. They come in threes." Sure enough. Two more explosions. She sang to him while I basically dipped him in a tub of water from armpits to feet.

All new parents will become poo-obsessed to a certain degree. Steve kept a log of his baby's poos and shared status reports with anyone who would listen, or who couldn't run away.

SAYING NO

I would rather deal with explosive diarrhea than negotiate boundaries with my family.

During the first week, there was a bit of a revolving door of welcoming friends and *mishpoches*. Like Jewish visitors everywhere, often people did not know when to leave. And we didn't have the guts to tell them.

It all came to a head when Eli was five days old. David was the recipient. He had come by every day and was always sweet and helpful. He always brought Gatorade and great snacks. On this day, he wanted to bring some friends by to meet the baby. We felt too depleted to be around people whom we'd never met. We wanted to be alone, and we finally said so. Bluntly. He was hurt. These friends were like family to him, and they hadn't met the baby yet. I told him that they could come to the bris (circumcision ceremony) three days from then. But three days was almost half of our baby's lifetime at that point.

———————————————————●———————————————————

To many people it is difficult to explain just how huge a drain on your tiny supply of human life force it is for them to come by and "hang out" for an unspecified length of time. So let me be clear to all prospective visitors: If someone you love has a new baby, do not hang out! Come, tell the parents how gorgeous their pointy-headed, wrinkly babe is — even though she might look like Mel Brooks — clean up, and get out. Those are better gifts than a cotton hat from Baby Gap. I hope someone will do that for you, and if they don't, show them this book.

———————————————————●———————————————————

SAYING NO . . . TO MOM
We had planned for my mother to stay with us for the first week. At one point on the third day, Janis went out to do an errand. Eli and I were konked out. An insistent tapping woke me. I crept

downstairs to see my sixty-three-year-old mother, standing on her tiptoes on a chair, scrubbing the light fixture in the living room like a whirlwind. Rest assured that that particular chandelier had not seen Windex in at least five years.

"My mother scoured every wall in our house. She vacuumed *under* the carpet. She said she was trying to make the air cleaner for the baby. We asked if she could come by once a week." – Netty

Besides delousing our dusty lights, during the days Lily would cook, clean, calm, and cajole with breathtaking kindness and ease. However, after a few nights, Janis and I realized that we didn't really need anyone with us overnight. When our son woke up he required me to nurse him, with Janis's help and cheerleading. Or he needed us to figure out how to get him back to sleep. These were assignments that we had to do ourselves, since they would be our job for the next year or so. So we told my mom that we really didn't need her to sleep on the lumpy futon in our living room any more.

This news, instead of being greeted with relief, was met with great sadness. My mother was dismayed that we didn't need her at night, that there was nothing "momlike" she could do for us. I tried to explain that she'd raised a self-sufficient daughter who was fine on her own. But she was inconsolable.

I felt horrible that I'd made my mother cry, when she was just trying to do something nice for us. So *I* was inconsolable. Poor Janis had a boatload of consoling to do. Other friends were envious of our situation. They had little or no support and we had so much. How could we be ungrateful? Yet, I knew we were right. Bonding as a threesome was the most important thing we could do. That and figuring out where our son's off switch was. (Eventually we realized there isn't one. You have to take out the batteries.)

● ● ●

Diapers: Cloth or disposable? There are pros and cons for each. Cloth is natural, non-irritating, better for the environment. On the con side: They need to be changed more often and require you to somehow scrape off the poop, and then launder them, or to pay for a laundry service. Disposables are easy, last longer between changings, and keep your baby more dry. However, they can be expensive, can contribute to landfill, and who knows what they're made of. In Toronto, there is a company called Small Planet that recycles disposable diapers and also offers all-cotton disposables, if you're environmentally conscious. That's the middle ground we went for. Most importantly, remember that for disposables, the front of the diaper usually has a picture on it, the back has sticky tabs.

● ● ●

8

The First Few Months

Put a Sweater on Him!

*To cope with the hormones that raged through my body, I developed
an alter ego. Someone I call Ferocita. In my imagination, Ferocita
looks like a maternal version of the Incredible Hulk, complete with
bulging muscles, breasts of steel, and an intact pelvic floor.*

By the time Eli was two weeks old, I developed the un-
shakeable belief that my son was the most supremely
gorgeous, glorious, and gifted baby you've ever seen.
And sadly, everyone else's child was a bit of a *mieskite*.

Eli stunned us with his special talents: the way he'd suck on his
toes, how he'd smile crookedly like a drunken sailor, the fact that
he thought he could stand up.

To provide a healthy reality check, Janis would remind me that
the skeevie baby things kept on appearing too, like: the nasal aspirator and all its snot-sucking implications; mucus-y, stringy poo
bits; and my hair in his diaper.

But by this point, even those grungy details registered as earthly
delights to me. I was changing drastically. Becoming something I
never imagined was in me. A mom.

BECOMING OUR MOMS

No matter how much we love our mothers, most of us have at one time chanted the incantation, "I will not become my mom, not I, not ever." Even if you have the iconic super-mom, there will be something about her that you will not want to pass on to your child. Because you are an intelligent and urbane sexpot, you cannot imagine slipping into your mother's old-fashioned habits.

Why on earth would you make your child wrap a damp cotton sock around their neck when s/he has a sore throat, for example? You'll leave the paper towel that lines your vegetable cooler where it is, even though it's certain to breed mould that will give your child lupus. I'm sure you've said to yourself, I don't care if my child finishes everything on her plate. In fact, we won't use plates. We'll eat with our hands in front of the TV. You vow that your innocent and impressionable babe will not be oppressed by the arcane anxieties or apathies that you inherited from your family.

I hate to break it to you, but it's going to happen. Your mother's phrases, songs, recipes, irrational fears, and the ridiculous solutions to them will pop out of your mouth willy-nilly. Even worse, some of them will work.

I personally thought I would be immune to this because I am temperamentally different from my mother, who claims to have, and have passed on to me, the Jewish Mother Gene (JMG). This gene causes characteristics of acute anxiety, fear for other people's safety above one's own, the compulsion to make sure one's child is eating enough and doesn't put something in their mouth that will give them ringworm, and a desire to shop on-line. Because my father is a strong and silent Scot, I hoped that I would inherit the recessive form of the JMG – something that might merely cause a mild heart palpitation when my child gets near a squirrel that is undoubtably rabid.

I have discovered through extensive research (i.e., phoning three friends) that there are two extremes of new moms: the earthy calm mom and the insanely anxious mom. Put another way, we have the "let him be" and the "put a sweater on him" mother. Mine was a "put a sweater on him" mom. I vowed that I would "let him be."

However, the odds were against me. It seems that there are many more moms on the "put a sweater on him" end of the continuum. For me it's been a rapid and slippery slide to the sweater side. It took no more than a few days before a whole world of anxiety opened up for me. I quickly developed a checklist of things that could go wrong. The following is an example of what passed through my mind, and will likely pass through yours, in the twelve seconds it took for Eli to start crying and be stopped by Janis:

"Is he hot? I think he's hot – oh he's cold, put a sweater on him, I have a couple in my pocket. Look, he has a rash, why does he have a rash? Maybe he's having an allergic reaction. It must be my fault. Probably it's something I ate. Why did I eat that Wheat Thin?! Do you smell that? Is that poo or a fart? Should I change him? I just changed him. Maybe I'll change him, oh I think it's passing. It *was* a fart. Why does he fart so much? What's wrong with him? He has no colon, probably. Where's his sock, where's his sock, where's his sock? Did you wash your hands? Did you use the antibacterial soap? I know it's creating a whole new race of super-bugs, resistant to all antibiotics, and we're all going to die wheezing and coughing in the dark, but get your skanky, *E. coli*, fecal-matter hands off the baby who has no colon! Okay, everything's okay, people have been having babies for millions of years. Put a sweater on him and let him be!"

As my son progressed through his first year, I hoped that my self-awareness and my ongoing wrestling with the Jewish Mother Gene would help to temper its influence. And often it did. Unfortunately, the JMG's twisted logic is at times irrefutable.

One day in the summer of his first year I was with a moms group that I refer to as The Groovy Yoga Mamas Group. We were hanging around in a nearby park that has a "splash pad," a concrete wading pool that is filled with cool water and maintained by the city.

The water is so cold that it shrinks your feet into red and wrinkly stumps in ten seconds flat. I was walking my then eleven-month-old son in, and he was screeching with joy, squatting in the water, splashing, trying to get me to take him deeper and deeper. I was resistant because I was freezing, and since I was cold, I kept taking him out of the water to warm him up. Every time I did this, he arched back and screamed. He obviously wanted back in. One of the other mothers said, "Why don't you just let him be? He's fine. It doesn't bother him." I had to explain patiently, in a very logical tone, that:

1) I'm Jewish. I'm not like those hearty Canadians who leap into the icy lake at their cottages on May two-four weekend with a beer in one hand and their inhibitions at home. I go into the lake so slowly that, yes, it does take all day, and I kvetch about the cold the whole time. I got this from my bubbe, who would stand and make "hooo hoo" sounds while moving at the pace of about an inch an hour in her ribbed and begirdled golden one-piece and her matching bathing cap with the appliqué flowers.
2) My son has to be cold because I'm cold. If he is not feeling it, it is because he has no nerve endings in his legs, and that is something else to worry about.

I carted Eli off to the sandbox where the only things I had to be concerned about were sand fleas, other bullying children, and hidden poop.

One of the less benign characteristics of the JMG that I had hoped to avoid was an acute awareness of all the evil in the world. Now, I simply cannot open the paper, watch the news, or listen to anything but the Oldies station. When I hear a tire squeal, I burst into tears, "What if a child was under the wheels of that car?!"

So here I am, acting like my mother in the most primal of ways. Should I embrace this phenomenon? Should we all call our moms and tell them how right they always were when they told us not to leave the house with a damp head? Or should we struggle against the pull of our mothers' and our mothers' mothers' DNA, lying in wait in our cells like a psychic time bomb?

You'll have to tell me. I'm too busy making sure that the baby keeps away from the microwave so he doesn't get irradiated.

MAMA BRAIN NEED SLEEEEP

Babies can poop, barf, and wail in a continually colicky fashion, and your instincts (be them JMG or not) will kick in and you will somehow cope. It is the sleep deprivation that makes you fall to your knees weeping, asking your partner questions like: "Will this ever end?" and "Who am I?"

You may be lucky. My sister's son started sleeping five hours at a stretch at two weeks. By six weeks, he was only getting up once or twice a night. By three months, he was pretty much sleeping nine to twelve hours. The universe must want her to have another child. Our experience was vastly different. So much so that we began physically to *crave* sleep. Sleep became our crack, our porn. We were obsessed. It was all we could talk about it or think about trying to get, as this e-mail from Janis can attest:

> "I'm beginning to dread the nights even as they are getting easier. This anxiety makes it so that I can't sleep. Instead, I read books about sleep. Which I never remember the following day. Sleep deprivation can do strange things to your mind and it makes me fragile and short-memoried."

The term *Mama brain* is used to describe this loss of short-term memory. Janis and I often wandered about like zombies, forgetting each other's names.

Other effects of sleep deprivation that we experienced were:

- loss of emotional perspective;
- all-day exhaustion;
- short-temper and . . . what was the other one? I can't remember. Stop bugging me! Excuse me, whatever-your-name-is, I think I need to cry.

When we were lucky enough to sleep, we dreamt about the cause of it all. Every night I had nightmares about Eli. Mostly they were connected to this little fact: it was down to *me* to keep him alive. Many parents I spoke to experienced the phenomenon of terrifying baby dreams involving losing, dropping, or forgetting to feed their child. My mother still remembers one that she had almost forty years ago.

"I dreamt that I left my baby amongst the vegetables on an outdoor stand at the local grocer's. I still remember the utter panic, running back and praying that the baby was okay and still there. And how the baby was there, quite calm, though a little perturbed, and that no one was paying much attention to the whole thing. I remember thinking, What will my father think of me now, I cannot even care for my child."

These dreams are based on the new anxieties of parenthood. There are so many details to remember that you're afraid you'll forget the most important one: the baby. To counter this, Kathy, a quick-as-hell actor and mother of two girls under three, gave us this brilliant insight: "Only try to accomplish one thing per day." In other words: *lower the bar.*

Before our babies were born, my pals and I all operated using long lists of tasks that we would check off throughout our day. Now a typical list is three words long: "get . . . to . . . bank."

The ever-wise and wiseass Patricia visited one day in the first few weeks. I admitted that I was feeling flabby and listless and foreign to myself. She said, "For the first three months, your job is to be the couch for your baby. Give in. Do nothing else. Just be the couch."

BREASTFEEDING PROGRESS

Besides, you have work to do that is much more demanding than returning your printer cartridge. Getting some fat on that baby.

As Eli and I got into the breastfeeding groove, I began to feel something that is called the "let-down." It happens as oxytocin (the hormone that is released by nipple stimulation) causes the muscles in your milk ducts to contract. It's an indicator that your milk is coming in and you better get that baby on the boob fast or you'll be wringing out a dripping blouse, sister. To me, let-down felt like intense electrical shocks tingling around my breasts and into my nipples, first the right, then the left. In the beginning it really bothered me. Soon I got to looking forward to it. It was my connection to my son's needs and my body's graceful rhythms.

As breastfeeding became easier, we had two challenges: getting our son onto a bottle and breastfeeding in public.

Take My Bottle, Please

Many books will suggest that you don't even attempt a bottle until the baby is six weeks old. The concern is that the baby may reject your breast in favour of the more consistent and faster flow of milk from a bottle. Eli was gaining enough weight, and obviously enjoying breastfeeding enough, that our midwives encouraged us to try to get him on a bottle of pumped breast milk at four weeks.

Ruth's sons got on the bottle no problem. Did I mention that she's perfect? So I thought that's how it would be for us. Not so much. Eli would cry and refuse to open his mouth when the bottle came anywhere near him. I swear he once gave Janis the finger.

I was advised to leave the house and let Janis give Eli the bottle so he couldn't smell me and want the breast. Someone else advised that *I* should be the one to give him the bottle, since Eli already saw me as the *food* source (nice). We were told to wait until he was really hungry so he had no choice but to take the bottle. We were told to try to feed him when he *wasn't* hungry so that he'd be less likely to cry.

At four weeks, Eli took his first bottle of breast milk. He drank two ounces. It had taken me forty-five minutes to laboriously pump that much using the electric cow-machine. This machine rhythmically sucks your entire breast into its maw, so that it looks like Playdough going through a vacuum. I eventually became so good at pumping that I would sit on my couch, the nozzle of the pump pressed into my breast, my legs crossed, and have business conversations with colleagues, "Well, you just tell that s.o.b. that he's your agent and he's working for you, godammit." I never flinched. I often pumped while watching TV. Maybe to remind me that I wasn't in a stable and I didn't chew cud.

> "I had to pump at work. I'd close the door and put the double-nozzled pump on each nipple and sit there as the 'rrr . . . rrr . . . rrr . . . rrr' sounds of the breast-pump confused and/or titillated everyone who passed by." – Laura

Once Eli took the bottle, we should have kept at it, giving him one small bottle a day. I was concerned that skipping a breastfeeding would cause me not to make the right amount of milk. Also, I guess we got cocky. It ended up taking him five months to accept a bottle consistently, and even then, he'd often only drink it from Janis or I.

By a few weeks in, I already needed a break, especially in the night, and I couldn't even begin to know how to take it.

Public Beware – A Breast!

Having breasts is like carrying a cooler around with no need for ice, water, or any actual food. Anytime, anywhere you can satisfy your child's hunger, which is good because in the beginning you never know when they'll be hungry. So, unless you plan on being shut-in for the next few months/years, you'd better prepare for breastfeeding in public.

My cousin Michelle vividly remembers getting numerous disapproving stares and clucks, mostly from women, at an upscale suburban mall called Bayview Village. Obviously, it doesn't take *that* village to raise a child. They'd starve to death.

Laura was told to "cover up" by some ass. Jackie, an otherwise unselfconscious new mom, timed her outings so she could nurse at home or in the car. Netty's brother walked out of a room she was in, whining, "Do you have to do that in front of me?"

I recently moderated a panel on queer parenting, which is just like regular parenting, but with better accessories. One of the two dads on the panel told me that he was often the only stay-at-home dad in a group of women. When he took his son to a swim class, all the women would relax at the end of the class and nurse their babies in the pool.

"Awwwww," I sighed sweetly.

He misinterpreted my sigh as a sign of commiseration.

"I mean, they're all sitting there, feet in the warm water, nursing away," he continued, starting to sound disgusted. "How would they like it if I whipped my dick out in front of them?"

I thought to myself (and later told people that I said): "The minute your dick starts making food for your baby, you can whip it out. Believe me, I won't give it a second look." In reality, I said nothing. I was speechless. What was a young, hip, gay dad doing with such an antiquated attitude toward breastfeeding? I was also flabbergasted by his equation of dick to breast because when I was nursing, I stopped seeing my breasts as sexual objects. I didn't understand how whipping one out and sticking my son on could make anyone uncomfortable. Even when he'd suddenly pop off and milk would come spraying out of my now-bawdily exposed, drooling nipple.

When Oprah did a show on motherhood, a woman on the panel said that when she and her husband would be in bed, she'd never let him touch her breasts. They'd been tugged at, yanked on, bitten, and worked hard all day. She wanted to hang a sign on them, "Closed for business."

Despite the fact that when you breastfeed, you are fulfilling the vital purpose of providing your child with sustenance, some people will get uncomfortable around you. It makes no sense. Sure, we can see people beating the crap out of each other on TV, gander at autopsy photos and live plastic surgery, but God forbid we catch a micro-glimpse of Janet Jackson's nipple. Oy.

To prevent any nipple sightings, there are lots of expensive nursing blouses that you can buy with discreet little slits in them. They work like spy-shirts, and they cover most of your breast while you nurse. There are great nursing bras (I recommend Bravado) that allow for easy, one-handed access. You can choose to nurse at a distance from people, or with a receiving blanket covering your baby's head and your breast.

I just did it openly, anywhere (including at a Tim Hortons with Janis's parents) and defied anyone to have a problem with it. I've been told that I had an aura of "I dare you to say anything, jerkoff." My sister openly nursed too, and she had size G breasts – that's right, G. When you're G, you cannot exactly be discreet. Just getting one of those girls out requires two hands. And then the baby's head is about three feet from your body, so what can you do? Just hope our uptight, out-of-date, hypocritical society can get the heck over themselves and let you feed your hungry, needy baby.

WAITING FOR THE WEIGHT

Speaking of hungry and needy, breastfeeding does make you thirsty and can make you ravenous. I was conscious to make sure I responded to these urges so that my baby had the most nourishing milk possible, and a mother who wasn't prone to passing out in midstep. So, dieting to get the pregnancy weight off was out for the first while.

Fortunately, people did warn me that immediately after having the baby, I would look like I was still six months' pregnant. But at six months the hard belly balanced out the booty and I looked kinda cute. After the baby, my stomach was a nine-month-pregnant stomach, but now all shmooshy. I could pull my skin out like an old balloon. And the rest of my body and face were puffy and/or saggy. The extent of my weight gain, now that I didn't have a huge belly to balance it, alarmed me.

Another lesbian couple just had their second child. Each woman has now carried a baby (nifty trick, huh?). When Jamea was leaving the hospital with the newborn that she had just birthed, a stranger came up to her partner, Dierdre, and congratulated her on her new baby. She looked at Jamea and said, "When are *you* due?"

Jamea smiled as she told this story, and then she began to cry. The tears were about more than just the shock of how she looked. Once again, a mother was blindsided by lack of information and false expectations.

I too anticipated that soon after having my baby, I would become me again. When I looked down at my legs, feet, and hands, they were foreign to me. It was as if they were behind a mist, all fuzzy outlines. I couldn't imagine how I would get them back.

The answer was: *pishing*. For the first week after the baby, it seemed my to-do list was: nurse, drink, and pee – often without warning.

Did you even know you had a pelvic floor before you got pregnant? You have one and it is very important. It stops you from peeing until you really want to. During pregnancy it's lazy due to the stretching and the hormones and the baby's head bouncing on your bladder. Immediately after the baby, mine went on strike. Anything made me pee. Laughing, sneezing, blinking.

However, I was grateful for the constant urination because in a few days, my swelling went down. When I looked in the mirror, I felt like hugging an old friend who'd returned from a long journey. The most welcome returnees were my feet. The veins and long toes, the bunions – those gnarly suckers looked good!

After the peeing did its work, I was still left with about thirty pounds of what wasn't baby or water. Common wisdom says that what took nine months to put on, will take as long to take off. Kathryn, my yoga instructor queen, told us that it takes two years for your internal organs to resettle back to their original positions. And sometimes they don't quite get there. In my case, a prolapsed uterus, separated stomach muscles, and slightly askew ribs and tailbone left me feeling like a broken teacup that wasn't quite glued back together properly.

In the first few weeks, Eli gained a pound a week, and I lost a pound a week. This is how it remained for much of the first few months. The pounds did not all "melt away" as Ruth promised me they would, and as they did for her . . . perfectly.

Back when I had broken the forty-five-pound weight gain in pregnancy and was over 170 pounds, I said to Janis that after the baby came (all's well), if I ever wasted my breath kvetching about putting on five pounds here or there, she was to slap me. Well, I kvetched. In the first few weeks and months, I noticed other women dropping the pounds while I stayed the same.

By week six, Netty was ten pounds *lighter* than when she got pregnant. Tammy lost thirty pounds in the first six weeks. (She also got pneumonia and shingles in her eye. I'd rather be fat.) My sister was back into her old jeans in eight weeks. Kathy in two. In fact, Kathy used to eat a huge, king-size President's Choice chocolate bar every day and the breastfeeding would just melt it all away. Sadly, I took stories like this to heart and tried them. So consequently, the pounds didn't melt off, they dripped off, slowly, like water torture. In effect, I lost very little in the first three months.

Instead, I became the couch: soft, cushy, easy to sink into. Until suddenly, the weight loss sped up.

Many mothers chock this phenomenon up to the baby suddenly being big enough to drink more milk, and thus speed up your already busy metabolism. It could also be due to the fact that you might be getting some exercise finally. Also, the baby's digestion really starts to settle at three months, so colic, midnight crying, and your inconsolable weepies diminish at that point. That reduction of stress could help you feel lighter too.

Like many nursing moms, I hung on to the last five or ten pounds until I was finished breastfeeding. By that point, many women forget what they used to look like and just keep the weight on. That, and the fact that it was near to impossible to work out like I used to, contributed to my body changing into a more mom-like vessel. Slightly looser, hippier, and rounder. Many people haven't noticed the change in me. I do, and it has got to be okay, because this body has worked very hard and deserves a break. From me.

STITCHES

One of the other most daunting things my body had to shed were the stitches in my Vajuj.

Because the hospital doctors did the stitching, Sara couldn't use the Midwife Collective's more sensitive ones, called Vicryl. So I got stuck with tougher, more wiry stitches that caused swelling and irritation in my tissues. I reacted badly to this, and my stitches became more and more painful each day. I wondered if I should have them taken out.

If you don't use a midwife, your first postnatal appointment with your OB might not be until six weeks. By then, your stitches will have dissolved. So hopefully you'll never have to experience them being removed.

(But, just to brag: our midwife came to our house to check on Eli and me on day one, three, and five. We went to the clinic for visits on day ten, fourteen, and after four and six weeks postpartum. That's seven checkups for the baby and me in the first six weeks. It was simply the most thorough and comprehensive medical care Janis or I have ever received.)

By our two-week visit with the midwife, my hospital stitches were more painful than they had been in the first few days. Sitting, walking, it was all becoming much more difficult, instead of better.

So, Sara suggested that she take them out. The tissues had knitted together by then, so the stitches weren't doing much anyway. We were still so blissfully in love with our midwife, that even when she said, "You may not like me after this," I didn't believe her. I once again assumed that some person would come with a thing. The thing that makes the stitches come out some other way.

Sara had to pull each stitch, hold it, clip it with some tiny scissors, then pull it out. Each one made me break out into a cold sweat. Before long, my legs were shaking and I was yelping out loud with each tug.

Following each snip, Sara asked how I was. Always the good girl, I told her I was all right and asked how she was. At one point she asked if I'd like to be done for the day and come back and finish up later. I asked how many more could there be? Janis's white face answered my question. I wished I had some Scotch and a bullet to bite on. Or just some Scotch.

After it was all done, I got to see the little buggers. They looked like tiny knotted bits of barbed wire. I was going to keep one, until I realized that I never wanted to see them again.

DEALING WITH TEARS – THEIRS AND YOURS

Many people told us not to fret the baby's tears. Confronted with our pale, drawn, wild-eyed faces, they assured us that since crying is the only way babies can communicate their needs to us, their desperate wails might be translated as, "Could you move your big head away from the window? I'm looking at something."

Eli used to cry from 5 to 7 p.m. every night. Janis and I would take fifteen-minute shifts. The TV would be on. Judge Judy would be telling someone that they better not think she's stupid, because she is not stupid. And one of us would be rocking and bouncing and cooing to a caterwauling six-week-old. Fifteen minutes would pass, and we'd switch.

When babies have what is commonly referred to as colic, they cry like this all day and night, often for three months. Our midwives admit that people don't really know what colic is, beyond a situation that is desperately painful for everyone to endure, and another dilemma that can only be solved by having it *end*. My mother still sharply remembers the mystery that is colic.

"The pediatrician put Daniel on rice cereal at one month. The baby immediately became colicky. It would last three months. The baby turned almost purple, tried to bend back almost double, and screamed and screamed. I did not connect it to the food. He cried, and I cried as I couldn't help him. I got an aggregate of two hours of sleep a day. I felt like walking death. I was afraid not to follow the doctor's feeding advice as he demanded that I add more and more foods, unheard of things like tapioca. He had no remedy for colic. One woman acquaintance of my mother had pestered me for years, 'So, when are you going to have a baby, when are you going to have a baby?' When I saw her again, she asked me how I was doing. I told her I was so tired. She replied, 'So, who told you to have a baby.'"

I refused to believe that Eli's crying was meaningless. I was sure that he *was* communicating complex thoughts to us through other

means, so therefore his tears must have meant that he was gen-
uinely upset.

I also believed that street signs were transmitting hidden messages to me (Squeeze Right means, yes, it's time to nurse on Right
Boob!), but lack of sleep will do that to you.

Then one day, I got it. I was in the kitchen holding Eli and trying
to do too many things at once, as usual. I kicked our pots and pans
drawer closed with my knee. Two glass pots banged together and
made a loud crashing sound. I didn't think it would bother our
snoozing fellow since he made demolition derby noises while
sleeping. He woke, had a huge Bob Fosse Jazz Hands startle reflex,
and burst into the most gut-wrenching crescendo of tears he had
expressed yet. He erupted in a loud wail, then was breathlessly
silent for what seemed like hours, then caught a huge breath, then
bawled again – louder.

I realized then and there that his keening was not always necessarily due to pain, to cold, to hunger. He still needed to be
responded to and comforted, yes, but he was *fine*. From that
moment on, I resolved to take a moment to suss out the cause of
tears and respond calmly.

Janis may disagree, but I think I've kept it up. And since becoming pregnant, I am always right.

FEROCITA!

One sleepless, absurd, reality TV–soaked night, I happened upon a
National Geographic special on grizzly bears. I learned a lot. Firstly,
that I'll watch anything. Secondly, when male bears wake from
hibernation, sometimes, in their ravenous hunger, they eat a stray
bear cub. Somewhere deep down, the Mama Bear knows this.
She has spent the winter hibernating, and her cubs have spent it
cuddled up next to her, suckling and growing.

In this documentary, there was a scene where a huge, lumbering male grizzly came too close to where a female was having a sip from a lake. Her cub must have been nearby because she *went after* that gigantic fellow, who was easily twice her size. She roared, her mouth unhinging to an impossible width. She threw herself at the male bear, and slashed him violently with her claws. She would not let up. He could have taken her head off with one swing of his massive paws, but he seemed to be stunned by her rage, taken off balance. He backed away, and I could almost hear him saying, "Whoa, lady, I just wanted a drink of water!" He quickly fled.

Most campers and wildlife experts have a healthy fear of mama bears, as well they should. People should also have a healthy fear of human mothers, because some of us have realized that anger is *good*.

This realization does not arrive gently. After Ruth's first baby came, she would get incensed with people who kept her on the phone too long. Robin punched a hole in her drywall. Victoria threw patio furniture around the front porch. Bev just lay on the living-room floor weeping and pounding the rug.

To cope with the hormones that raged through my body, and for the sake of my relationship, I developed an alter ego. Someone I call Ferocita Fiurosa. She was a close relation of the "fer fuck's sake" lady. I needed her so that I could abdicate all responsibility for my actions in my full-on mama bear fury. In my imagination, Ferocita looks like a maternal version of the Incredible Hulk, complete with bulging muscles, breasts of steel, and an intact pelvic floor. Instead of turning green, Ferocita burns a tasteful lilac.

Ferocita's head has snakes and scales and big red-rimmed eyes (and really skanky breath). She is not alone in the world. Many mothers develop super-human alter egos.

"If I feel my child is threatened, my head twists all the way around and I breathe fire." – Bev, mother of two

A defining appearance by Ferocita occurred when Eli was about a month old. Janis and I were invited to a friend's house for dinner. I thought that Eli might need to nurse before we went, but we were a bit late, so we left our house anyway. Ten minutes into the trip, Eli started crying in his car seat. The high-pitched, rhythmic, unrelenting newborn hungry cry. My teeth ground themselves to points. My irises turned pale lilac. The buttons popped on my nursing blouse. The legs of my maternity pants (that I hadn't even remotely got out of yet) ripped provocatively to expose bulging quads upon which there suddenly and miraculously was no cellulite. The elasticized front of my stretchy jeans rippled with a six pack. My skin tone started to match Eli's little purple hat with the kitties on it. Diane was no more. *Ferocita* was hunkered down in the passenger seat. Growling.

"How could you care more about being late to our friend's than Eli's hunger?" Ferocita spewed at Janis as we burned through an amber light about two minutes from our destination. "Who cares if we're late? Who cares if we never eat again? Are *you* hungry, is that it? Who cares?! I don't. I don't care about our friend's feelings. I don't even want to be her friend any more. She doesn't get it. You don't get it. The baby's hungry, dammit. Stop the car now, or I will stop it for you!"

Ferocita gives the finger to people who don't move aside for her stroller on the sidewalk, to people who smoke on patios, who get too close to the baby on an elevator, who try to pick him up without first disinfecting themselves. Ferocita is the kind of mother who would not only lift a VW off of her child, but would twist it into a pretzel and wrap it around the driver of that buglike German deathtrap. Ferocita has no fear, knows no mercy, and feels no repercussions.

Ferocita is great to have on hand for dealing with bad drivers, insurance companies, old girlfriends of your partner, and scammy telemarketers. But her effect on friends and family can be regrettable.

Before having the baby, I, like many women, was not exactly comfortable with my anger. Well, now with Ferocita, that's over. You know that moment during an argument where each person admits they were wrong? I don't do that any more. It would be pointless, since, as I mentioned, I'm always right.

The result is that fights with Janis last longer, are more intense, and veer close to the edge of something. Like with the great love that we feel for our child, we are at times overwhelmed, afraid, and at a loss. We take a lot of walks. After which we enjoy a lot of yummy making-up. Ferocita has made our devotion to each other more intense too.

No one, but no one, better even *breathe* funny around a Ferocita and her kid.

"I took my son to Ikea to get some baby crap. I had him in the little cart and he was doing great. Happy, chatting to himself. Kinda loudly. A woman passed by and rolled her eyes at us. I stopped her, 'Excuse me, did you just roll your eyes at my kid?' I demanded. We argued until she left the scene. About ten minutes later, the eye-roller found us again and she said, 'I'm sure you're happy to know that your child will grow up to be a loudmouth like you.'

'Well, I bet you're thrilled that any kids of yours will be *skanks* like you!' I yelled back." – Aara, mother (bear) of one

As Aara told this story, she pushed up her sleeves to show us her pumped, heavy-baby biceps and her razor-wire tattoos that seemed to cry out, "Me, you – parking lot!"

One night in the first few months, Eli, Janis, and I were all in the tub together. We were playing with a bath toy, a floating plastic primary-coloured Noah's ark, complete with nondescript two-by-two animals and a round male and female stick-in shipmate. Janis innocently asked me, "What was Noah's wife's name?"

"She didn't have a name," I answered, "she was called Noah's wife."

"Goddamn patriarchy," she muttered, and handed Eli to me.

"Yeah, fucking patriarchy!" I said, hot tears of fury springing from my eyes for the world my son was to enter.

I carried my baby from the tub, holding his wet, warm, soft body in my arms, wrapped in a towel, ready to be diapered and feet-pyjama-ed. Ferocita was pounding hard in both of our chests, just below the surface, primed to protect Eli from all manner of social injustices.

Ferocita-type feelings come from hormones, yes, but they also come from the pure and tender ache to protect that vulnerable little being. When Eli sleeps, an aura surrounds him of such delicate sweetness, it breaks my heart. Many parents talk of wanting to bottle their baby's smell, to keep the gentle luscious essence of them safe forever. I trust that Ferocita will do what she can to make that happen. Or bust some heads trying.

RELATIONSHIP REALITY CHECKS

You know how in your relationship, although you may have numerous fights, you really are only having the same one fight over and over? Sometimes it may come out like: "Don't tell me how to drive," but it's usually about a core issue between you. Due to lack of sleep, these hot buttons – painful, deep, ancient – will become flash points after the baby.

Added to that, the overwhelming love and sense of responsibility for your child (the Ferocita factor) will undoubtably make you shift your priorities away from each other to the new baby. This can be very disconcerting to you both but, rest assured, it is really common. Janis described a feeling that she'd better help or get the hell out of the way. That Eli and I were in a circle of two. Luckily, she often created a similar circle that overlapped with mine.

Although we were great teammates, we didn't always agree on how to cope with Eli's mysterious needs. In those moments, we had to negotiate whose instinct would be heeded. As stressful as those disagreements may have been, I'd rather have too many chefs (even if they're coming at each other with a loaded Moulinex) than a big old empty kitchen. In those first months, I don't think either of us would have handled being home totally alone with our child with much grace.

We always say that Janis conceived of our child (because it was her dream to have him) and I bore him (because I have the jaggedy labia to prove it). So we were committed to maintaining as much equity in parenting as possible.

Since we are each extremely privileged to work at flexible vocations, Janis and I agreed to both be home part-time for the first nine months (this stretched into fourteen months). We ended up living on less, but we never went out, so we never spent anything. If Janis had any hesitancy about not working, it disappeared as she became more and more intoxicated by our child. I was happy not to take much work and, coincidentally, people were happy not to offer it to me. Hmm . . .

Janis and I were not the norm among the other new parents that we met. We discovered that most dads went back to work pretty soon after their child was born, even if they had the resources not to. In *Misconceptions*, Naomi Wolf describes all these equitable feminist couples she knew who suddenly flipped into traditional male/female gender roles when their babies came. She states that she is mystified and horrified by this trend. But she also says that her husband went back to work after two weeks. He got a new job.

As a result of this kind of role-splitting, many working partners miss out on significant bonding opportunities, including some that are not so delightful, like night-feedings.

> "When my husband and I went to bed, he put in earplugs. That left me to take care of all the crying, feeding, tummy aches, and midnight diarrheas alone. He explained it by saying that he had to work the next day." – Ellen

Too many of us have swallowed the line that work outside the home, work that brings in the dirty lucre, is much more important than raising a healthy child. After all, no one gets paid for mothering, although we'd probably all agree that we've never worked harder in our lives. The injustice of this makes me insane.

> "I was dragging my son, Adam, down the stairs in a subway station in his stroller. I'd bumped the stroller down the stairs wheel by wheel, trying to balance my bag and his stuff. No one offered to help me. A man passed me, winked, and said with a kind of jovial grin, 'The things women have to do, huh?' I said, 'Well, we wouldn't have to do it if you guys would help.' The man kept on walking. I yelled after him, '*That's* why we have to do it!'" – Victoria

I overheard a mother telling her friend that her husband is really good at taking care of his own needs, while she can't seem even to identify hers: "Eric really needs to work out on the weekends, and I'm too tired to argue." In my fantasy, Ferocita barged in to that conversation, carried that poor, sunken women to a gym, let her take a whirlpool, and have an hour to herself. In that time, Ferocita would observe Eric as he cared for his baby, and point out all the areas of his body that have started to sag: "Hmm, a goatee can't hide those jowls, Eric," Ferocita purred in my mind.

I don't want to give the impression that I am just blaming the partners here, though some, like Mr. Earplugs, deserve it. A lot of moms can't seem to trust their partners to find their own way to comfort and feed their child. They can't let go, and they don't encourage their partners to bond and be responsible. "Oh, you know men, they just can't manage to feed a baby. Why even try?" Baloney.

It does feel great to have a little one totally attached to *you* and wanting your attention all the time. Your baby cuddles you, softly touches your face. It is sensual and terribly fulfilling. But if you don't let go, and let your partner comfort this child, you will all regret it. Everyone will lose out. So, let go, Mama, let go. You'll be letting go their whole life.

Ultimately, those first months are so fleeting that if there's any way that you can swing it, *why not both share them?*

CIRCUMCISION

There are some moments that aren't fleeting enough. Our son's circumcision occurred in our living room at 7:45 a.m. on his eighth day as a separate being.

Prior to the service, Janis and I got together with the female mohel, or mohelet, a GP named Dr. Rochelle Schwartz. She was unfazed by my phone message wherein I warned her that we were an interfaith lesbian couple with a father who was recognized and Jewish. There were three sets of grandparents that needed to be acknowledged, and we had a really big dog.

Rochelle is a warm, bright feminist doctor who believes that bringing a community together to witness parents pledge commitment to education, enlightened spirituality, and love can only serve a child well. She also has a great laugh. She jumped on board.

Rochelle had developed a pain protocol. An hour before the bris, she coated the baby's penis with a fingerful of topical anaesthetic, followed by a needle of freezing. Eli was then given baby

Tylenol and sugar water, and also a tiny sip of ceremonial super-sweet Kosher wine, after which I swear I heard him say, "Feh."

The ceremony began. Janis, David, and I were terribly anxious. We propped each other up, the three of us gripping hands and elbows, openly sobbing. My parents sat by the table where the mohelet had her big goblet of wine, prayer book, and surgical instruments. Eli had to be held down with his legs open, which is what started his crying. Most mothers retreat to a corner and barely watch at this point. But Rochelle called me over when Eli's crying started to escalate. Janis stepped back, clearly distraught, wanting no part of this ritual, her face red-rimmed and crumpling.

The actual circumcision was over fast. Foreskin cut, wrapped in gauze to be buried later in the backyard. Odd, how keeping the placenta was considered ooga-booga feminist, yet the whole community jumped on the "let's bury the foreskin somewhere special in the backyard, but nowhere where a dog might pee on it" bandwagon.

The baby's cries became sharper after it was over. The mohelet nodded to me, as per the prearranged signal. The nod meant, "You can take the baby and go upstairs to try to calm him by nursing him, while I finish up here with the prayers, and the welcoming to the community, and the wine drinking." The nod, of course, meant nothing to me in my shock, so the mohelet actually had to give me a little nudge and a "Go nurse him. Go take him. Go."

Janis and I took the wailing baby upstairs. I nursed him while Janis stroked his head. Someone knocked at the door. I had asked that no one come up after the bris, in case Eli was upset. I motioned for Janis to tell them to go away. But it was Ruth.

"Diane, it's me. Let me help."

I let her in. She sat opposite me and in soothing tones repeated over and over that it was all right, he was going to be fine. Slowly, Eli's tongue came out and he started sucking in between sobs, both his and mine.

In the living room, the ceremony was winding down. All the mothers in the room had tears in their eyes, and most of the fathers were green around the gills. We heard the cheer go up, like breaking glass, "*Mazel tov!*" The mohelet started the singing and everyone slowly joined in, rising to a chorus of barely remembered and certainly not understood Hebrew words, in a soup of ancient, cherished melody.

Back in Eli's room, I apologized abjectly to Janis and promised that if we had another son, we would never do this again. Now, like so many things said in those days, including, "I still remember the pain," my conviction is fading.

SLEEP STRATEGIES – NOW WHAT?
Did someone say, "Fading?"

We'd had our little guy for a few months now. Since other parents had babies who slept without waking to feed at night, we naturally assumed that ours would too. We obsessively looked for patterns, but before they're three months, there's very little consistency in anything: napping, eating, pooping, smiling. You are bound to get frustrated if you expect anything but chaos.

> "Well, for the three nights before last, Eli woke up and was unable to go back to sleep at around midnight, 2:30, 4:00, 5:30, 6:00, and 7:00 a.m. We were walking around like two stoners, forgetting each other's names. 'You are? . . . And I know you because? . . .'" – Excerpt from our sleep journal

In response to all this, we read every book there was on sleep. The strategies varied from feeding in bed with you on demand, and only putting them down to sleep once they are totally conked out, to letting them cry and making sure you put them in their crib while they're still awake so they can get *themselves* to sleep.

A whole book could be written about the practical pros and cons of these approaches. (Please see the reference section in the back for my totally biased summary of some of the more popular sleep books.) We were certainly not comfortable letting him cry himself to sleep at this age so we shared the night wakings. Sometimes I'd nurse him and sometimes Janis would comfort him. The idea was to slowly wean him off of the idea that every time he woke up, he would get the breast. Sadly, the operative word in our case was *sloooowly*.

It wasn't easy for me to resist breastfeeding him in the night. I often had to wrestle Ferocita to the ground. Each time Janis went into Eli's room with a pacifier, I wanted to go over there and grab him from her arms. "He's hungry," Ferocita Fiurosa bellowed in my head, "everyone get outta the way!" I struggled to ignore Ferocita's command. "Janis and I are in this together!" I mumbled through gritted teeth. "She's doing this for all of us, and *he* is fine!" I won, and Ferocita slunk back under my skin. For the moment.

A neighbour and her partner had a strategy of three nights on, three nights off. She would do all the night feedings for three nights in a row, letting him sleep through. Then he would take over. She said that a one-night-on, one-night-off pattern never really allows you to recover from sleep deprivation. This strategy implies that your child will take a bottle at night. If you can get that sorted out, it might be a nice way not to lose your marbles.

Some babies cluster feed – feed every hour or less for a few hours right before bed, in effect filling their tanks and allowing them to sleep longer. We tried to convince Eli of the wisdom of this tactic, but he would not budge. Unlike me, he could not accept that eating when you're not hungry, eating just because the food is there, is a *fantastic* idea.

The cruel irony is that if and when you do get your baby to sleep uninterrupted through the night, *you* may forget how to. Like many of my sadsack, worrier friends, as soon as Eli started sleeping longer than two hours at a stretch, I continued to wake up.

Before I got pregnant, I was able to sleep through most things and sleep almost anywhere. Janis loves telling the story about how I once fell asleep at a party. Standing up. The party was in full swing, and a friend was regaling us with a story about her trip to a yoga retreat in the Bahamas. The only thing more boring than doing yoga all day is hearing about it. I did indeed lean against a doorframe and fall asleep while the party raged around me.

I used to be called "the ten fifty-seven girl" because I'd never be able to stay up for Letterman. Those days are gone, and I miss them. I, like many moms, have had to recondition my brain to remember what it is like to sleep uninterrupted (or unaware of every cough, sigh, or mutter) through the night. To this day, if I am sleeping and something disturbs me, I have a post-traumatic stress reaction. I'll take anything to help me get back to sleep: milk, chamomile tea, antihistamines, Gravol, sleeping aids, a bonk on the head. I told Janis that in this one realm, she is with a junkie.

Then there's Victoria. She said that all the night-waking has turned her into a person who is able to fall asleep any time, any where, no matter how long she's been awake.

My wish for you is that your little one sleeps long and easily so you never have to find out which of the above you are.

SEX?
Don't be ridiculous!

Some books will say that you *can* have sex again after six weeks. After all, your Vajuj isn't bleeding any more, so let's hup to it.

When Netty's son was nine weeks old, Steve asked her if she would like to have sex. She asked if he would like her to stick her finger in his penis.

Reasons why you may not want to have sex, or even masturbate, for quite a while longer than the stupid arbitrary six weeks:

- Rampant libido-suppressing hormones: the effect of which is affectionately dubbed "drier than desert."
- Exhaustion: the minute you are horizontal, the only person you want to make love to is Mr. Sandman.
- Sore breasts that also ooze.
- The ever-active Mama brain. Numerous and random thoughts may make you feel like sex should be the last thing on your list: "Has anyone done the laundry? I have sixty-two new e-mails. Shouldn't we eat instead? I wonder what's on TV. Shh, was that the baby? Why would you even want to have sex with me?"
- Totally warped body image or, in my case, an accurate body image whose sexuality I was not comfortable displaying.
- "Primary maternal preoccupation" (an actual psychological term that sounds pretty spot-on to me). If all you can think about is your baby, with immense love and fear, how are you supposed to let go and do something just for you and your partner? Soon you'll *want* to figure this out. Right now, you don't have to even try.
- The fear that sex could result in another one of these darling angels before this one learns to distinguish sun from moon. I know people *do* get pregnant again soon after the first, my own parents included, but I never said they were all that bright.

When you are ready for sex again, you'll know. But you might need your partner to be persistent, and to help you to turn your Mama brain off. You may not feel like it right now, but you do have needs.

BECOMING A JOINER

Moms group — noun. A bunch of people from whom you desperately seek advice. People to whom you never would have listened in your previous life.

Have I mentioned that I'm not exactly a joiner? Step classes make me break out in hives. Even spontaneous communal gatherings like red lights get my heart pounding. Yet, by the time Eli was a few months old, I became desperate for the company of other moms. I needed specific anecdotal advice from live human beings. "Has yours ever banged himself repeatedly in the head with a phone?" I needed to know that other moms didn't know what they were doing either.

The moms groups became a real source of comfort, but at the beginning, I felt very outside, and perhaps a little judged:

> "Today I met with the Midwife group. And I felt so out of place and insecure. I felt different than them. Is it because Janis and I are doing this together? Is it because I'm older and an artist? Is it because I feel like an ignoramus? I had no idea what a 'saucer' was — some sort of toy — whatever it is, we don't have one for Eli. They know all the words and actions to all the songs! They all speak the same language. Or was I just worried because Eli hadn't nursed much and didn't seem to want to nurse for more than 3.5 seconds when he was there?" — Excerpt from my journal

I am so glad I stuck with it. Despite the fact that our parenting philosophies vary wildly, some of the women I met there have become real friends. Which is good, because some of our "real" friends have become scarce. They seem not so interested when we share the kinds of details one can only delight in at a gathering of parents: "Can you believe it? This morning, my son stared at my alarm clock for seven minutes straight! Wait, shh, maybe he'll do it again."

Plus, the snacks at a moms group are always superb.

Please go ahead, eat those nachos while you analyze your babies' many different kind of smiley faces. Now, after you have a brownie for dessert, you *might* think of getting a little exercise. With so much to do, it becomes very easy to neglect your body's basic needs. Like the need to talk to someone without saying the words "one sock . . . two sock." These may not seems like priorities to you right now. I bet they are to your partner.

After the baby, many husbands or partners are physically not so different from how they were before the baby. They may have sympathetically put on a few pounds with you (which is the decent thing to do), and they may be sleep-deprived, but their bodies inside and out are very much the same. So they can imagine getting back to how they were nine months ago. They can see a light at the end of the tunnel. Therefore they often have a deep need to work out or have sex or grasp on to some sense of how they *used* to be.

For many birth moms, we are completely changed inside and out, and have been since we conceived. "How we used to be" is not an option. We can't even see the tunnel, much less the light at the end of it, so we don't understand (and may resent) our partners' physical needs.

In this instance, I empathize with your partner. (I *like* you, but s/he is right on this one.) Even if you don't feel like it, getting some sort of exercise in the first few months is a great idea. You may be depressed by what you can't do yet, but you will amazed with what you can. And you will be without the baby for an hour. You need that, Mom, you really do.

It might be easier to do it with a group of other moms who are in the same slightly rickety place that you are.

When Eli was six weeks old, I went back to yoga classes, now called postnatal yoga, at the Yoga Space. It's a superb concept. You bring your child with you, and the instructors and volunteer baby-minders pick them up when they fuss so that you can relax and do your class.

The instructors were aptly excited to meet Eli. And boy, did he ever do me proud. While other babies cried throughout the class, he lay on his back on my yoga mat, swiping and cooing at my fingers, at the sun creeping across the wall, and the tingle of the Buddha bells.

At the beginning of the first class, the instructor, Sasha, warned me to take it especially easy. Although I felt better, I sensed that my body was like a jigsaw puzzle that had been shaken up a bit: some pieces were in place, and some were stuck to the underside of the box.

We began by lying on our backs and breathing. I did this so well that I became extremely confident about tackling the next task: tightening up my overextended core muscles. We were told to sit up. I asked my stomach muscles to contract and get me to a sitting position. After a few minutes with no answer, I realized that my abdominals must be on another call. I lifted my head, but could not roll up any farther. I dialled my stomach muscles again. The line just rang and rang.

About ten weeks later, things were much different. I returned to my first boxing class. I remembered how to skip, to punch, to do a man's pushup again. It was amazing! However, I did discover that when I did a jumping jack, I peed. I felt warm liquid run down my leg, and I thought I had gotten my period. (The common wisdom is you won't get your period until you finish breastfeeding. Mine came back after ten weeks.) Then I realized the liquid was still coming. I ran to the bathroom. I had peed my pants. So like every good mother, I adapted. No more jumping jacks. For a few more months, I did gliding jills instead.

Despite the steepness of my recovery curve, I was delighted by how much the muscles in my body did remember. During those moments, I could almost forget the miraculous thing my body had recently done. Until I sneezed . . . and everything dropped.

I DROPPED THE BABY

At some point you may accidentally do something that makes you want to call the Children's Aid Society on yourself. The baby is fine, but you may want to lock yourself away in a dark room and thrash and wail that you are an unfit mother, that this is all too much for you, and who the hell thought you were adult enough to take full responsibility for another being anyway?

"I was in the park with the girls on my way to the Sears Portrait Studio to get their pictures taken. I was taking them both off the swings, and as I half-turned to warn Josie not to walk in front of the swings, *bam*, Phoebe got clobbered by walking in front of another swing. Every mother in the park gave me that look, not the 'Oh you poor thing with two little ones how do you manage it?' look, the 'Jesus, lady, haven't you learned yet or is this just your nanny's day off and you're giving it a shot for once?' look. I felt horrible. Plus, I can't take them to Sears for a picture until the damn bruise goes away." – Kathy, mother of two

Many mothers don't drop their babies so much as – in their sleep-deprived haze – helplessly observe them as they fall. Or, if you're me, accidentally knock the softest part of their skull into the corner of a cupboard.

"Today I went to Costco with Henry. He fell backwards out of the cart. Of course, he landed on his head." – Ruth

"I left my daughter in the stroller on our front porch while I opened the door to the house. I didn't realize that the whole porch must have been built on a slight slope. I was trying to find my keys in my overstuffed diaper bag, and suddenly I see the stroller, as if in slow motion, roll down all the stairs and flip over onto the sidewalk!" – Loretta

"I have bumped Jordan. Quite a few times actually. I did it today trying to get him into his car seat. I hate when it happens. He just starts to cry and looks at me like I am from hell. Why did I do this to him? . . . Thankfully he is made of plastic." – Laura

Ah, the car seat. Occasionally, my son likes to stiffen his compact little body into a board to prevent me from getting him seated. I end up trying desperately to bend him while vainly struggling with straps and clips. I'm always afraid that I look like one of those "caught-on-tape" moms. The ones who say they just "snapped." I wish they'd invent a car seat with suction, so you could just bring your child anywhere near it and they'd get sucked into the appropriate safety position.

As a mother, you're always multitasking. Recently, at a swimming class with Eli, I watched as a mom changed her wet, wriggling baby, tried to dry herself, and open her locker door, "You know what women should grow during pregnancy?" she blurted. "A third arm!"

It's true. We get all that wiry body hair, the dark tummy line, why couldn't we grow something that we could actually use later on? Mind you, then we wouldn't acquire the skill of being able to pick our purses up with our toes.

But back to dropping. I too have dropped, stopped, and wailed. The first time it happened was when Eli was about seven months old and my parents were over for a visit. He had just started eating in his high chair. Ann Lamott, in her wonderful book *Operating Instructions*, describes feeding her son as "spackling." You put some food in the hole, then use a spoon to scrape off all the gunk on the sides of the hole. Then you refill the hole.

My parents had spent most of the day playing tirelessly with Eli. I, however, was pooped. Eli had just spent the last ten minutes using his pablum to disprove the laws of physics. I needed to get him out of his high chair, clean the cereal off the floor before it dried and stuck like barnacles to a barge, and get him to bed.

Usually my post-spackling procedure was as follows:

1) take tray off high chair;
2) unstrap baby from high chair;
3) take baby to sink and wash him;
4) clean tray and floor and walls and fridge and appliances and ceiling and own hair.

But in my exhaustion my inner list got messed up. I did the following:

1) take tray off high chair;
2) unstrap baby from high chair;
3) clean floor and . . .

At that moment, Eli leaned forward and reached for me. There was no tray to stop him or straps to hold him back. We all heard a sickening *splat* as he landed face first on the floor. He did not know enough to use his arms to protect his head. He did not know that no one would catch him. And I failed him. I let him fall. I could hear his innocence packing up and leaving.

I scooped my wailing baby up. I kept it together until I got him upstairs and into nursing position, but when Janis closed the door my floodgates opened. I sobbed and sobbed, silently so as not to further upset him. I stroked his face and told him how sorry I was, that I would always protect him in future.

Janis came downstairs and told my parents that everyone was all right and that they didn't need to stick around. My mother, a Ferocita Suprema, refused to budge, "Maybe the baby is okay, but what about *my daughter?*" she demanded as she puffed up to twice her size.

Dropping the baby is generally harder on the mother.

"I was pushing Adam in our big SUV-type stroller with the Mag wheels. The big back wheel got caught on the curb or something and the whole thing fell sideways onto the street with Adam in it. He hit the dirt face first. All of our stuff was splayed in the road. I ran around in a panic shushing Adam, who was now wailing, trying to grab all my gear. Then a guy came along and started helping me. I felt like I had to explain to him that I was a good mother, my stroller was possessed, maybe there was a bump in the sidewalk. The guy then told me the story of the time that his stroller flipped right over and his daughter landed on her head. The saga of this nice guy's misfortune calmed me enough to get me home and bawl myself to sleep. All night I watched Adam, shaking him every twenty minutes to make sure he didn't have a concussion." – Victoria

My mother has many stories of us falling, jumping, and (horrors!) wandering away. My mother's friend Linda says that in the event a child wanders off, you should check the direction of the wind. The children always run with the wind; it's easier.

After three kids, my mother has a poetic perspective on the whole dropping thing.

"The event can go from the ridiculous to the tragic. And that is the fear that wakes you in the midst of night, and washes over you. I think that perhaps the hardest thing for a mom is the eternal vigilance, and the taking of actions to eliminate any possibilities. And how, sometimes, things happen anyway. The amazing thing about children, besides the fact that they are often made of rubber, is that they forgive you everything! And love you still." – Lily

How can they not forgive you? You're adorable!

Cute Things You New Parents Do

- forget simple words, like *egg*;
- fall asleep at 8:30 p.m., while your partner is kissing you – in the middle of the kiss;
- pick things up with your toes like a primate;
- wipe up diarrhea, snot, pee, and vomit like it's spilled milk while talking on the phone, changing your child, and remembering the word *egg*;
- start to understand what people mean when they say there is nothing more awesome than this.

———•—•—•———

Do whatever makes you comfortable to try to get your baby to sleep. No one else's agenda or timing is right for you or your child. Your baby will eventually sleep on their own. In fact, one day they will try to put a lock on their bedroom door.

———•—•—•———

9
A View from the Bridge

The great secret I have been let in on is that most new parents are a bit over the moon with love. It's amazing we can function at all.

A s each stage passed in Eli's newborn development, we'd look back on it with the sensation that we were standing high up on a bridge. From that vantage point, we'd say, "If we only knew then what we know now." If only we could have had a view from the bridge.

What I'm realizing now is that the bridge never ends. You don't ever get all the way across, but you do experience unimaginably resplendent vistas on the way. Each phase of your baby's growth is so new and dazzling that you are motivated to keep stepping forward. Unlike on a real bridge, you can't go back. Your child is past it and moving on, and so are you. You are actually doing it.

YOU *ARE* HANDLING IT

When Eli was eighteen months, I had a terrible dream. My son was made of salmon. He wasn't *a* salmon, his body was made of cooked salmon instead of skin and bones. In the dream, I was watching over him desperately because he was so light and flaky. At one point in the dream, I had to run into a building and get his sling to carry him, so I asked a friend to hold him. And she handed him off to Keanu Reeves. Keanu was someone I acted with when I was a teenager, and he was an electrifying actor but, I would suspect, not so great with salmon-skinned babies.

Sure enough, Keanu dropped the baby into a river. I got back in time to see Eli fall. I leapt into the water, and although I am bigger and stronger, I couldn't catch up to him. He floated over a swell and was gone. I could only flail my arms and breathlessly watch him float away.

I knew I had to kill myself.

I woke from the dream weeping and told Janis that she is never to let anyone but her watch our baby. Ever. Then I told her that I felt incompetent as a mother. I was not capable of dealing with the emotional and psychic stress of having a baby. She reminded me of all the times in this journey that I've said, "I'm backing out!" When we were inseminating, after I started having terrible nausea, when I started pushing him out. She replayed all those nights when I sobbed, "He's so cute!" into her armpit. His inescapable adorableness, in his little yellow sleeper, would break my heart into a million pieces, and completely overwhelm me.

All those times I was sure that I could not handle what I was in fact handling. I now know that I am a good mother. I am responsible, excellent at multitasking, very aware of potential benefits and hazards in his path, patient. The flipside of my anxious and obsessive nature is an eagle-eyed caregiver. But the thought of him in pain or distress is enough to kill me. I find it terribly hard to tolerate. When he goes into Grade 7 (all's well), I'll probably have to be on Xanax.

Fortunately, I'm not the only one. The great secret I have been let in on is that most new parents are a bit over the moon with love. It's amazing we can function at all.

When my son was a little over a year, I did a workshop of a new play with a local actor, Ron White. Ron is about fifty, a compact, grizzled tough guy, who tends to play brooding psychopaths. He's confident, driven, and successful. I've always been a little intimidated by him. I found myself walking side by side with him at our dinner break.

We strolled in silence for a few minutes. And just as I was worrying that, since becoming a mom, I didn't have anything interesting to say to anyone, he reached into his wallet and pulled out pictures of his new baby.

"Can you believe how great it is, Flacks? I had no idea. This is what all those parents are talking about!"

I tried to get a word in, but Ron went on, "The joy, huh, Flacks? It makes sense of life, doesn't it?"

This feeling is similar to falling in love. You know that phase when you use any excuse to say your new flame's name, "Speaking of global marketing, Brad has the cutest moustache . . ."? Now, any flimsy pretext to talk about your child, and you're off. "Yeah, I agree about the mapping of the humane genome. Did I mention that Madeleine knows all the words to 'Wheels on the Bus'?"

SEX AND THE MOMMY

When my Groovy Yoga Mamas Group got together a year later without our kids, we desperately needed to talk about three things: fighting with our partners, sleep, and sex.

At one point, after the wine arrived, we suddenly looked around the table and realized that everyone had truly become a mother. People who are, as Hannah said, paraphrasing *The Big Rumpus* by Ayun Hallyday, like leaky ships in a big ocean. We wave to each other with love and hope and recognition, as we constantly bail our boats in order to stay afloat.

We checked each other out. We needed an aerial view. To compare how we were doing in the average scheme of things. The first subject was sex. We didn't have an official agenda, or anything. Someone at the end of the table just whispered "sex" and everyone dropped the topic that was so important a moment ago (jolly jumpers, spit up, food allergies, hand-foot-and-mouth disease) in order to chime in, "Are you talking about *sex?*"

Yes. The guilty secret that no one was having any. We gathered some statistics:

- 5 out of the 7 of us had sex an average of 4 times in the last two years.
- 2 out of the 7 of us had sex somewhat regularly. Freaks.
- 3 out of the 7 reported the mystifying experience of suddenly having a surge of horniness out of nowhere that lasted from a week to a month and then, just as suddenly, screeched to a grinding halt.
- 7 out of the 7 of us reported feeling like we were just not the "same" physically and we were self-conscious enough about that to be reticent in initiating sex.
- 2 reported saying these seductive words to their loving bedmate: "Stay on your side!"

We looked at the stats, sighed, and decided that the best strategy now was to order more calamari.

Slowly, we started to tell stories about our children and our experiences as parents. I was most relieved to hear that other women were also experiencing relationship upheaval.

"BRIDGING" THE RELATIONSHIP

Dura Mater: (*Latin, tough mother*). *The outer membrane protecting the spinal cord and brain.*

I once asked Janis what was the single biggest way that she thought I had changed since having our son (besides the droopy boobs). She told me that I was tougher. This toughness is crucial to help you survive being a mother, but what does it do to a relationship?

In the winter when our son was a year and a half, he got a disgusting virus after revolting bacterial infection, and passed them all on to Janis and me. Ear infections, followed by flus, bronchitis, and the dreaded and recurring explosively purging stomach flu. Near the end of this marathon, I hit the wall. Janis went to work and Eli suddenly got much worse. As I rocked him and let him puke down my back and stick his germy fingers in my eye, I felt that I couldn't take another round.

Janis was planning to get home to relieve me around six-ish. Time began creeping ever slower from four o'clock on. I counted the minutes. (I am sure that I saw 5:13 more than once.) Then Janis got a call at work from her brother, asking for her help with something important. She figured she could do it all: work, see her brother, and still be home before the baby fell asleep. She didn't make it.

What she did instead was spark an irrational and sustained bout of sarcasm on my part. Each morning I'd come up with a new put-upon-wife cliché, "Have a nice day at work, sweetie. I'll just be hanging out with a bottle of Scotch and my friends from *Canadian Idol*. Maybe your brother will ask if you could help him feed his cats. So come home after that. The baby will be in bed and I'll be drunk." Janis had a sense of humour about it. Until she didn't. So then I stopped.

The complexities of trying to balance work and home life are daunting. They create real, uncompromising obstacles to resuming a formerly healthy, empathetic relationship.

"He wanted to go to his parents' and cut their grass for them! After I'm home with the baby all week long! I could have killed him. Just 'cause his dad had a stroke . . ." – Tanya

"The dog woke us up between the two times that the baby woke us. I told my husband that it's time to put her down. She's three years old . . . but I can't take it any more. He loves that dog more than me!" – Jeannie

"My partner and I have had more fights in the first year of our child's life than we did in the previous eleven years together. No one tells you about this." – Victoria

Many women confided turning to their partners at various points in that first year and asking plaintively, "Do you even like me?" When their partners embraced them and said, "I *love* you," they would push on with, "But why?"

So, here are some suggestions that other people offered to help us pass through this difficult transition in our relationship:

- *Go away for a romantic overnight.* Try not to get into a fight the instant you hit the hotel room. Try not to call home eight times an hour. Try to have sex, but don't act like you're trying. If nothing else, sleep in. The first time we were away from Eli for the night, I got my period, Janis got a cold, and we got into an irrational row about the room service. But we did it *alone.*

    One word of caution – if you're nursing, bring your breast-pump! Or you'll wake up with throbbing, bursting, painful rocks for boobs.

- *Do not talk about the baby after s/he has gone to bed and you are finally alone with your spouse.* Do not panic when, if you do not talk about the baby, there are huge lulls in your conversation. Instead, you can both use these lapses to catch a little shut-eye.

- *Have a date night once a week.* A special night that you can reserve for just you two. Do not put it off for any reason, like exhaustion, sick baby, sick babysitter, good TV on at home, major deadlines at work, getting in a fight about the above.

  Victoria suggested a date night during the *afternoon* instead of the evening. After getting the baby fed, washed, and to bed, you are too pooped, hungry, and overstressed to enjoy a game of pool.

  The first time we went out to a movie, we felt like we'd been living in a cave, wherein we had been raised by wolves. Everything seemed too bright, loud, and shiny. We considered turning back, but bravely trudged up the moving stairway in the big building-with-stores (that's *escalator* in the *mall*, for those of you who don't speak wolf).

  We clutched each other's arms and took seats in the aisle. The movie was that godawful *Lord of the Rings*. It was unspeakably loud, and the battle scenes were relentless. I kept my cellphone on the whole time, clutched in my sweaty palm, so I could grab it instantly if my mother called. (We would only leave Eli with her for the first while.) I bawled to Janis that I was a bad mother. Why did I leave my baby when he needed me?

  When we returned home the baby was a bit hungry, but I let him nurse and he was fine. Moreover, Janis and I got to look into each other's eyes again. Even if that look was, "How can we make these big computerized ghouls shut up!"

Here's some of *our* relationship strategies that might work:

- *Be demanding.* As Victoria said to her man, "You're a really good dad, but *I* need you as well."

- *Get a therapist.* Someone who will come to your house while the baby's napping and who will give you drugs.

- *Be gracious and tender with each other.* Touch your partner when s/he is sleeping.

- *Try to see the humour in your behaviour.* You are a mother. Therefore, technically you are a lunatic.

- *Tell the truth, no matter how irrational.* Be open with your emotions. Don't be afraid to fight, cry, and let it all out. Your partner is going to feel the cold front anyway.

- *Drink. More. Wine.*

- *Don't worry.* You are *both* working hard to adjust to this new life and create an environment that nourishes your baby. You may end up discovering that it is very sexy to watch your partner figure out how to handle life.

If you have found that your relationship is experiencing disconnect, be comforted that you are not alone! With time (and sleep) the bond does return, often in a richer, deeper form.

I am lucky to have a partner who is incredibly attuned to my needs. Frankly, I am lucky to have a partner. I do not know how my single-mom friends did it and still do it. They are marvels.

AND *YOU* KEEP ON A' CHANGING
Besides a tougher you, a child often enhances your tender side. What a gift in our cynical, over-industrious world.

"You know, before I had my daughter, I was a thousand times more cynical and I cried almost never, I couldn't stand 'sucky' anything – and that child has *ruined* me! I am now officially one of the biggest sucks on the planet – I am a card-carrying member of the Hallmark Suck Club! Kids do that to you. I can't stand the little bastards!" – Sass

We are unapologetic about our new-found sucky delight in our beautiful, magnificent, exceptional, multi-talented child – you should see a picture, *k'nein a hora*!

If you choose to nurse, the biggest *physical* change you will experience are the breasts. Zoe described her breasts now as like old paper bags. They're thin and greasy from too much use. Mine look like they're constantly running away from each other, and careening down the outside of my rib cage. So, I bought a good bra.

One of the changes in my *personality* that occurred to me around Eli's first year was a loss of lightness. One day, Janis took me out for a walk so we could have a "talk." Yoiks, I was braced. I knew Ferocita had been pushing it a bit. Instead Janis pointed out that I seemed to have lost my silliness, my ease. I hadn't done any schticky sound effects, or even a pratfall, in months. She missed me.

Soon, levity started to rush back. No amount of soul-searching, therapy, or watching Madeline Kahn movies precipitated this. The reason that I started enjoying myself and others again was because we were finally getting sleep.

Eli began sleeping through the night when he was about a year old. He did it himself, when he was ready, just as Janis's mom predicted he would. We now readily acknowledge that we didn't so much train him to sleep as help him to get where he was already going.

As Eli's schedule finally began to gel, we started going out with friends again, and, to our surprise, we became a source of information for other new moms. We tried not to judge, or to give too much unsolicited advice. We failed utterly.

At one baby shower, as our gifts of a sling and some baby wipes was being opened, one of the assembled guests shouted out, "Give them some advice from the world of experience!"

Flashing through all the words of wisdom that were imparted to us, through all the changes we'd weathered, and the crazy new love we were sharing, I shouted back, "Wipe the hands first, then the bum. Not the other way around."

And Janis added, "Good luck!"

K'nein a hora, ptoo ptoo ptoo.

• • •

Every child is different. Some are "easy babies" that allow you to resume your life almost as it was. You see these parents sipping beers on patios as their child coos quietly in a high chair. We did not experience this. Other children may require you to make more drastic changes to what you assumed was your life. You may eventually find great freedom in the truism that it's not about you any more. In the meantime, be patient with yourself and each other. And keep repeating, "Just seventeen more years . . ."

Seventeen fleeting, astounding years.

• • •

References

THE SLEEP BOOKS: A BIASED SUMMARY

What to Expect in the First Year by Arlene Eisenberg: Common-sense solutions, lots of age-old advice, offering many options and info, not specifically committing to any one. Like the Liberal party. And me.

Solve Your Child's Sleep Problem by Richard Ferber: Let 'em cry, but check on them. But don't touch them. But talk to them. Try to do so cheerily. Grind your teeth into nubs and get into huge fights with your partner. Many people swear by this method. I hear that if you can stick it out, you may get some needed sleep.

Secrets of the Baby Whisperer by Tracy Hogg and Melinda Blau: Like Ferber, but instead of leaving them, you stay and pick them up until they stop crying, then put them back down on their own again, then pick them up when they start crying again, then put them down. Exhausting, but a viable middle ground. Needs a good strong British temperament and back.

The No-Cry Sleep Solution by Elizabeth Pantley: Do everything in your power to teach them to fall asleep on their own, while still nursing and holding them. Support for the notion, "Whatever works."

The Baby Book by William and Martha Sears: Nurse them in your bed, listen to their needs. Carry them in a sling like a kangaroo. Trust that eventually they will want their own room – when they're twelve. Forget what your partner's body feels like next to yours for a while. This places a lot of burden on the nursing mother, and can't work real well if you are a working mom. But it made tremendous sense to Ferocita, who roared in my ears to respond to every cry. NOW.

GENERAL PREGNANCY BOOKS
What to Expect When You're Expecting by Arlene Eisenberg, Heidi
   E. Murkoff, and Sandee E. Hathaway
Birthing from Within by Pam England and Rob Horowitz
The Hip Mama Survival Guide by Ariel Gore
The Big Rumpus by Ayun Halliday
The Girlfriends' Guide to Pregnancy by Vicki Iovine
Operating Instructions by Ann Lamott
The Baby Book by William and Martha Sears
The Birth Partner by Penny Simkin
Misconceptions by Naomi Wolf

OTHER SOURCES OF INFORMATION
www.babycentre.com
Telehealth Ontario 1-866-797-0000
www.smallplanetinc.com

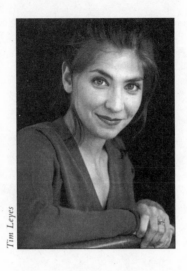

Tim Leyes

Diane Flacks enjoys picking things up with her toes and talking about herself in the third person. She has written and acted in theatre, TV series, and film across Canada, the U.S., and Britain. She has appeared in productions as diverse as *A Midsummer Night's Dream*, the *Royal Canadian Air Farce*, *The Vagina Monologues*, and *The Kids in the Hall* show (for which she was Emmy-nominated as a writer). Other published work includes her hit solo show *By a Thread*, and the play *SIBS* (written with Richard Greenblatt), as well as numerous magazine and newspaper articles, and internet publications. She lives in Toronto with her partner, Janis, and their son, Eli. This is her first book. Visit www.dianeflacks.com.